THE POWER OF HEALING HERBS

OVER 75 HEALING REMEDIES FOR VARIOUS AILMENTS

G. V. BLOOME

Disclaimer:

I am an herbalist, not a licensed medical professional.

The information provided in this book is

Intended for educational purposes only and it is not

Intended to replace medical advice or treatment

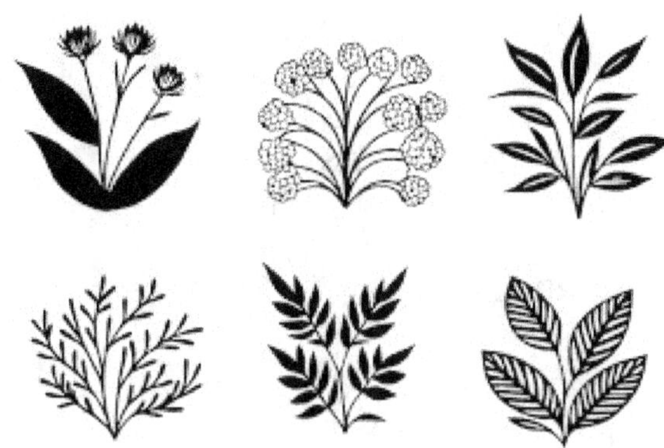

INDEX

TOOTHACHE
HEARING PROBLEMS
BAD BREATH
HAIR LOSS
ASTHMA
GALLSTONES
MOTION SICKNESS
EPILEPSY
WARTS
STYES
HAY FEVER
BRONCHITIS
LOW BLOOD PRESSURE
INTESTINAL PARASITES
DANDRUFF
VARICOSE ULCER
DYSPNEA
INFERTILITY
ENDOMETRIOSIS
PROSTATE
OBESITY
SCIATICA
SEASONAL ALLERGIES
HEPATITIS
RESPIRATORY DISTRESS
STROKE
CANDIDA
TOURETTE SYNDROME
OSTEOPOROSIS
PARKINSON'S DISEASE
ALZHEIMER'S DISEASE
NERVOUS SHOCK
RHEUMATIC DISEASE
EXCESSIVE SWEAT
ARTERIAL COMPRESSION
RESTLESS LEG SYNDROME
URINARY TRACT INFECTION

GASTROENDERITIS
HIGH CHOLESTEROL
MENINGITIS
ARTHRITIS
WHOOPING COUGH
FOOD POISONING
HEART ATTACK RECOVERY
CHRONIC STRESS

"It is health that is real wealth and not pieces of gold and silver..."

Mahatma Gandhi

Herbal Remedies and Their Significant Role in Our General Well-Being: Why Choose the Natural Path to Health?

In a world increasingly dominated by synthetic medication and fast-paced living, many of us are turning back to our roots. The age-old practice of using herbal remedies is enjoying a renaissance as people seek natural alternatives for better health and wellness. We find ourselves surrounded by a plethora of options for self-care, and exploring the realm of herbs offers us an opportunity to reconnect with nature and our own innate healing capabilities.

The Holistic Approach: Connecting Mind, Body, and Spirit

When we think about health, it's essential to adopt a holistic approach. This perspective recognizes that we are more than just physical beings; our emotional, mental, and spiritual health is intricately woven together. Herbal remedies align with this holistic philosophy by offering solutions that support the body, mind, and spirit rather than simply focusing on one aspect of our health.

As Mahatma Gandhi once said:
"It is health that is real wealth and not pieces of gold and silver..."

This quote beautifully encapsulates the idea that our true riches lie in our health and well-being, which can be influenced profoundly by the natural tools at our disposal.

Understanding Herbal Remedies

Herbal remedies encompass a wide range of plants and natural substances used for healing purposes. These remedies have been employed for thousands of years in various cultures, from Traditional Chinese Medicine to Ayurvedic practices in India. The resurgence of interest in herbal treatments has sparked a wealth of information about how these plants can improve our health.

Popular Herbal Remedies

Here are several widely-used herbs and their purported benefits:

- **Echinacea**: Often utilized to boost immunity and ward off colds and flu.
- **Ginger**: Recognized for its anti-inflammatory properties and benefits in digestion.
- **Turmeric**: A powerful anti-inflammatory and antioxidant, praised for promoting joint health and combating chronic diseases.

- **Peppermint**: Frequently used to ease digestive discomforts and enhance mental clarity.
- **Chamomile**: Valued for its calming effects and effectiveness in promoting sleep.

Each of these herbs offers unique properties that can contribute significantly to our overall well-being.

The Benefits of Choosing Herbal Remedies

We might wonder why we should choose herbal remedies over conventional medicine. Here are several compelling reasons:

1. Fewer Side Effects

One of the most significant advantages of herbal remedies is the lower incidence of side effects. Many pharmaceutical drugs come with a long list of potential adverse effects, while herbal alternatives often boast a gentle nature, particularly when used appropriately. While herbal remedies are not devoid of side effects, they tend to be milder and less harmful than synthetic options.

2. Holistic Healing

Herbal medicine emphasizes treatment of the entire person — body, mind, and spirit. For instance, chronic stress can manifest as physical ailments; herbal solutions often address the root cause of these issues.

By choosing to integrate herbal remedies into our health routine, we embrace a holistic healing process that aligns with our natural make-up.

3. Rich Nutritional Profile

Many herbs are packed with essential vitamins, minerals, and antioxidants that strengthen our overall health. For example, dandelion greens are a powerhouse of nutrients, including vitamins A, C, and K. By incorporating herbs into our diet, we enhance our nutritional intake naturally, providing our bodies with the tools they need to thrive.

4. Empowerment and Connection to Nature

Picking up a bottle of herbal tincture or drying herbs in our kitchens creates a tangible connection to nature. The process of understanding, sourcing, and preparing these remedies empowers us to take charge of our health. As we engage more with the natural world, we foster a greater sense of well-being.

5. Sustainability and Accessibility

Herbal remedies can often be grown in our gardens or sourced locally, making them an accessible and sustainable option. This local sourcing leads to healthier ecosystems and promotes community connections. We cultivate not just our health but also our relationship with the earth.

Seeking Professional Guidance

While herbal remedies present a promising pathway to health, it's crucial to approach them with informed wisdom. We should always consult healthcare professionals—preferably practitioners experienced in herbal medicine—before embarking on a new treatment plan, especially if we are taking other medications.

Frequently Asked Questions (FAQs)

Q: Are herbal remedies safe for everyone?
A: While many herbal remedies are safe for general use, certain individuals—such as pregnant women, nursing mothers, and those with specific health issues—should exercise caution and consult healthcare professionals.

Q: How long does it take to see results from herbal remedies?
A: The timeline for seeing results can vary widely depending on the individual and the specific herbal remedy being used. Some effects may be felt almost immediately, whereas others may take several weeks to manifest.

Q: Can herbal remedies interact with prescription medications?
A: Yes, certain herbs can interact with pharmaceutical medications. It's critical to consult with a healthcare provider to prevent adverse interactions.

Q: Where can I find high-quality herbal products?
A: Quality herbal products can often be found at health food stores, herbalist shops, and reputable online retailers. It's essential to choose products that undergo rigorous testing and provide transparency about sourcing.

Q: How can I incorporate herbal remedies into my daily routine?
A: Incorporating herbal remedies can be as simple

as brewing herbal teas, adding herbs to our meals, or even using essential oils in our self-care routines.

Start small and gradually explore the vast world of herbal healing. Choosing the natural path to health means embracing the wisdom of traditional herbal remedies that have stood the test of time. By adopting a holistic approach, we honor the intricate connection between our body, mind, and spirit. Remember, each time we opt for an herbal solution, we are not only nurturing our health but also reconnecting with nature in a meaningful way. By using these herbal remedies, we empower ourselves to take charge of our well-being while fostering a sustainable connection to the earth. As we venture into this natural realm, let's keep in mind that the path to health is not solely about eliminating disease but about nourishing the richness of our lives.

Below you will find over 75 herbal recipes for various mental and physical distresses. There are not only herbal remedies and the detailed descriptions on how to make them, but the information about each particular disease, its description including symptoms and causes, along with the best herbal recipe to either treat that specific illness or profoundly relieve its symptoms.

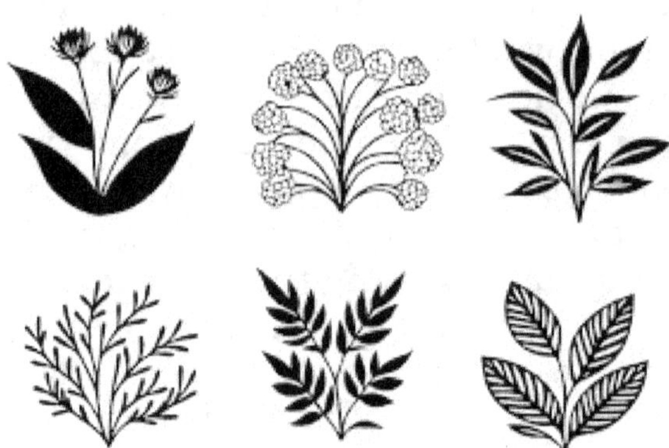

1. Herbal Healing Recipe for Common Cold

As the seasons change and the air turns crisp, many of us find ourselves battling an unwelcome foe: the common cold. Symptoms like a runny nose, sore throat, cough, and fatigue can take a toll on our daily lives. While over-the-counter medications are available, turning to nature can provide effective relief without the side effects often associated with pharmaceuticals. The information below will guide you through an herbal healing recipe that can help soothe cold symptoms and support your immune system.

Understanding the Common Cold

The common cold is caused by various viruses, leading to inflammation in the respiratory tract. Symptoms usually appear 1-3 days after exposure to the virus and can last for about a week. While there is no cure for the common cold, herbal remedies can alleviate symptoms and promote a speedy recovery.

Ingredients for Our Herbal Cold Remedy

For our herbal healing recipe, we will utilize the following powerful ingredients, each chosen for their unique therapeutic properties:

1. **Echinacea**: Known for its immune-boosting capabilities, Echinacea is often used to prevent colds and reduce their duration.

2. **Elderberry**: Packed with antioxidants, elderberry can help reduce inflammation and support respiratory health.
3. **Ginger**: This warming spice has antiviral and anti-inflammatory properties, making it a great ally in combating cold symptoms.
4. **Honey**: Not only does honey soothe a sore throat, but its natural antibacterial properties aid in recovery as well.
5. **Lemon**: Rich in vitamin C, lemon boosts immune function and adds a refreshing taste to our remedy.
6. **Cinnamon**: Adding a touch of warmth, cinnamon helps in decreasing inflammation and supports overall health.

Herbal Healing Tea Recipe for Common Cold

Ingredients

- 1 tablespoon dried Echinacea root
- 1 tablespoon dried elderberries
- 1 tablespoon grated fresh ginger (or 1 teaspoon dried ginger)
- 1 tablespoon honey (or to taste)
- Juice of 1 lemon (freshly squeezed)
- 1/2 teaspoon ground cinnamon
- 4 cups of water

Instructions

1. **Prepare Your Herbs**: If you are using dried ingredients, ensure they are fresh and of

good quality. If using fresh ginger, peel and grate it.

2. **Simmer the Mixture**: In a medium saucepan, add the Echinacea root, elderberries, grated ginger, and water. Bring the mixture to a gentle boil, then reduce the heat and let it simmer for 20-30 minutes. This allows the flavors and medicinal properties to infuse into the water.
3. **Strain the Tea**: After simmering, strain the mixture using a fine mesh strainer or cheesecloth into a large glass or pitcher.
4. **Add Remaining Ingredients**: Stir in the honey, lemon juice, and cinnamon. Adjust the sweetness to your liking.
5. **Serve and Enjoy**: Drink warm to help soothe your throat and clear your sinuses. You can store any leftover tea in the refrigerator and reheat it as needed.

Tips for Maximizing Effectiveness

- **Hydrate**: Drink plenty of fluids alongside this herbal tea to stay hydrated, as this can help thin mucus and ease congestion.
- **Rest**: Your body needs energy to fight off the virus, so ensure you get plenty of rest.
- **Steam Inhalation**: Consider doing steam inhalation with hot water and adding a few drops of eucalyptus oil, which can help clear up nasal congestion.
- **Maintain a Healthy Diet**: Include foods rich in vitamins and minerals, such as

fruits and vegetables, to further support
your immune system.

Final Thoughts

While the common cold can be bothersome, an
herbal healing tea can be a naturally effective way
to relieve symptoms and support your recovery.
The combination of Echinacea, elderberry, ginger,
honey, lemon, and cinnamon creates a soothing
blend that not only tastes great but also
nourishes your body at a time when it needs it
most.

Remember to consult with a healthcare
professional if your symptoms persist or worsen.
Stay healthy, and may this holistic approach
guide you to feeling better soon!

Happy sipping!

2. Herbal Healing Recipe for Stomach Ulcers: Nature's Remedy for Digestive Comfort

Stomach ulcers, or peptic ulcers, can be a painful and debilitating condition. They occur when the protective lining of the stomach is compromised, leading to sores that can cause discomfort, bloating, and indigestion. While traditional medicine often recommends medications to manage symptoms, many people are turning to herbal remedies for relief.

Understanding Stomach Ulcers

Before diving into our herbal recipe, it's important to understand what stomach ulcers are and their causes. These sores can be caused by a variety of factors, including:

- Overuse of non-steroidal anti-inflammatory drugs (NSAIDs)
- Infection with Helicobacter pylori (H. pylori) bacteria
- Excessive alcohol consumption
- High stress levels
- Smoking

Symptoms often include a burning sensation in the stomach, bloating, belching, nausea, and in severe cases, vomiting blood or experiencing dark stools. If you suspect you have an ulcer, it's crucial to consult a healthcare professional for a proper diagnosis and treatment plan.

Herbal Healing Recipe: Soothing Ulcer Tea

This herbal tea combines ingredients known for their stomach-soothing properties. It incorporates *licorice root, slippery elm, marshmallow root,* and *chamomile.* Together, these herbs may help promote healing, reduce inflammation, and alleviate discomfort.

Ingredients

- 1 teaspoon of dried licorice root
- 1 teaspoon of slippery elm powder
- 1 teaspoon of marshmallow root
- 1 teaspoon of dried chamomile flowers
- 4 cups of water
- Honey (optional, for taste)

Instructions

1. **Combine the Herbs**: In a mixing bowl, combine the dried licorice root, slippery elm powder, marshmallow root, and chamomile flowers. Mix them thoroughly to ensure an even blend.
2. **Boil the Water**: In a saucepan, bring 4 cups of water to a boil.
3. **Brew the Tea**: Once the water is boiling, add the herbal mixture and reduce the heat. Let the tea simmer for about 10-15 minutes. This allows the active compounds to infuse into the water.

4. **Strain the Tea**: After simmering, strain the tea using a fine mesh strainer or a cheesecloth to remove the plant material.
5. **Sweeten (Optional)**: While the tea is still warm, you may add honey to taste if desired.
6. **Serve**: Pour the tea into a cup and enjoy!

How to Use

Drink this soothing herbal tea 2-3 times a day, especially before meals or when you feel discomfort. The tea can help coat the stomach lining, reduce inflammation, and alleviate symptoms associated with ulcers.

Benefits of the Ingredients

- **Licorice Root**: Known for its anti-inflammatory properties, licorice root may help protect the stomach lining by producing mucous and preventing further irritation.
- **Slippery Elm**: This herb creates a gel-like substance when mixed with water, which can coat and soothe the digestive tract, potentially speeding up the healing process.
- **Marshmallow Root**: Similar to slippery elm, marshmallow root also forms a protective layer over the lining of the stomach, aiding in relief from irritation.
- **Chamomile**: Renowned for its calming effects, chamomile can help soothe anxiety and digestive upset, making it a wonderful addition to this healing blend.

Final Thoughts

While herbal remedies like this soothing tea may provide some relief from the symptoms of stomach ulcers, they are not a substitute for professional medical treatment. Always consult with a healthcare provider, especially if you experience severe symptoms or if you are currently taking medications. In addition to herbal remedies, consider making lifestyle changes that may help prevent ulcers from worsening. These include avoiding spicy foods, reducing stress, quitting smoking, and limiting alcohol intake. Embracing a healthy diet rich in whole foods can also support overall digestive health.

Enjoy this herbal tea as part of your wellness routine, and may you find comfort and healing in nature's bounty! Remember, your health is your wealth—take care of it naturally and wisely.

3. Herbal Healing Recipe for Migraines: Nature's Remedy

Migraines can be debilitating, impacting our daily lives, productivity, and overall well-being. While traditional treatments are often utilized, many people seek natural remedies to alleviate their symptoms. One such approach is the use of herbal remedies.

Understanding Migraines

Before diving into the herbal remedy, it's crucial to understand what migraines are. Migraines are severe headaches often accompanied by other symptoms such as nausea, vomiting, sensitivity to light or sound, and even aura sensations (visual disturbances). Triggers can vary widely from person to person but often include stress, certain foods, dehydration, hormonal changes, and environmental factors.

Herbal Allies for Migraines

Nature offers a plethora of herbs known for their therapeutic benefits. The following herbs have been traditionally used to provide relief from migraines:

1. **Peppermint (Mentha piperita)**: With its cooling and soothing properties,

peppermint can help ease tension headaches and improve blood flow.

2. **Ginger (Zingiber officinale)**: Known for its anti-inflammatory properties, ginger can help reduce nausea and has been found to be as effective as some traditional migraine medications.

3. **Feverfew (Tanacetum parthenium)**: This herb has been used for centuries to prevent migraines and may reduce the frequency and severity of attacks.

4. **Lavender (Lavandula angustifolia)**: Known for its calming properties, lavender can help relieve stress and tension, often triggers for migraines.

5. **Willow Bark (Salix alba)**: Often referred to as "nature's aspirin," willow bark can help reduce pain and inflammation.

Herbal Healing Recipe: Soothing Migraine Tea

Ingredients:

- 1 teaspoon dried peppermint leaves
- 1 teaspoon dried feverfew leaves
- 1 teaspoon dried ginger root (or ½ teaspoon fresh ginger, grated)
- 1 teaspoon dried lavender flowers
- 2 cups boiling water
- Honey or lemon (optional, for taste)

Instructions:

1. **Combine the Herbs**: In a teapot or a heatproof container, mix the dried

peppermint leaves, feverfew leaves, ginger root, and lavender flowers.

2. **Add Boiling Water**: Pour the boiling water over the herbal mixture. Cover the container with a lid or a towel to retain the heat, allowing the herbs to steep.
3. **Steep**: Let the tea steep for about 10-15 minutes. This duration allows the active compounds in the herbs to infuse into the water.
4. **Strain and Serve**: After steeping, use a fine mesh strainer to remove the herbs from the liquid. Pour the tea into a cup.
5. **Optional Enhancements**: If desired, add honey or lemon for taste. Honey can also contribute to soothing sore throats sometimes accompanied by migraines, while lemon adds a refreshing twist.
6. **Enjoy**: Sip on the herbal tea slowly. It's best to enjoy this tea while in a calm, quiet space—a perfect environment for relaxation.

Additional Tips for Managing Migraines

While this herbal tea can help alleviate migraine symptoms, consider these additional lifestyle changes and practices to manage migraines effectively:

- **Stay Hydrated**: Dehydration can trigger migraines, so drink plenty of water throughout the day.

- **Identify Triggers**: Keep a migraine diary to identify potential triggers and manage them accordingly.
- **Practice Stress Management**: Techniques like yoga, meditation, or deep-breathing exercises can help reduce stress levels.
- **Limit Caffeine and Alcohol**: Both substances can be migraine triggers for some individuals, so monitor your intake.

Herbal remedies can offer a natural and gentle way to manage migraine symptoms. This soothing herbal tea combines several approach curated to promote comfort and relaxation. As with any natural remedy, it's essential to listen to your body and consult with a healthcare professional, especially if you experience frequent migraines or are currently on medications. Embrace the healing power of nature, and may your journey toward relief and wellness be filled with peace and comfort. Remember that a personalized approach is often the most effective, so feel free to experiment with different herb combinations to find what works best for you.

Cheers to your health!

4. Herbal Healing Recipe for Chest Congestion: Breathe Easy with Nature's Remedies

Chest congestion can be a distressing condition, often accompanied by discomfort, coughing, and difficulty breathing. While modern medicine has its place, many people turn to herbal remedies for relief. Nature provides a plethora of plants known for their ability to soothe respiratory issues, reduce inflammation, and promote overall lung health.

Understanding Chest Congestion

Chest congestion occurs when excess mucus builds up in the airways, making it difficult to breathe and often leading to a persistent cough. This condition may arise from various causes, including colds, flu, allergies, or respiratory infections. By utilizing natural ingredients, we can create a soothing remedy that not only alleviates congestion but also supports overall respiratory health.

Our Herbal Healing Recipe: Eucalyptus and Thyme Infusion

Ingredients:

- 2 tablespoons dried eucalyptus leaves
- 1 tablespoon dried thyme leaves
- 4 cups of water

- 1 tablespoon raw honey (optional, for taste)
- Lemon slices (optional, for added flavor and vitamin C)

Instructions:

1. **Preparation**: Begin by measuring out your dried eucalyptus and thyme leaves. Eucalyptus is well-known for its ability to break up mucus, while thyme has antibacterial properties that can help fight respiratory infections.
2. **Boiling Water**: In a pot, bring 4 cups of water to a rolling boil.
3. **Infusion**: Once boiling, remove the pot from heat and add the dried eucalyptus and thyme leaves. Stir gently and cover, allowing the mixture to steep for about 10-15 minutes. This will enable the herbs to release their beneficial oils and compounds into the water.
4. **Strain**: After steeping, strain the infusion into a teapot or heatproof container to remove the solid herbs.
5. **Add Sweetener and Lemon**: If desired, stir in a tablespoon of raw honey for sweetness and drizzle in fresh lemon juice or add lemon slices. Both honey and lemon can enhance the flavor and provide additional soothing properties.
6. **Enjoy**: Sip the herbal infusion slowly while it's warm. This soothing drink can be consumed 2-3 times a day for optimal relief.

Why These Ingredients?

- **Eucalyptus Leaves**: Eucalyptus is renowned for its decongestant properties. The essential oil contained in the leaves, eucalyptol, works to loosen mucus and make it easier to expel. It also has anti-inflammatory and antimicrobial properties.
- **Thyme**: Thyme is not only savory in your dishes but also a powerful ally against respiratory ailments. It contains compounds that can help relax the muscles of the respiratory tract, making breathing easier while its antimicrobial properties can help fight infections.
- **Honey**: This natural sweetener has soothing qualities that can help reduce throat irritation caused by coughing. Honey also has antimicrobial properties, providing an extra layer of protection against infections.
- **Lemon**: Rich in vitamin C, lemon supports the immune system. It also adds a refreshing flavor to the infusion, making it enjoyable to drink.

Additional Tips for Relief

While sipping on your herbal infusion, consider these additional strategies to ease chest congestion:

- **Steam Therapy**: Inhaling steam from a hot shower or a bowl of hot water can help loosen mucus in the chest.

- **Stay Hydrated**: Drinking plenty of fluids can help thin mucus, making it easier to expel.
- **Maintain Humidity**: Using a humidifier in your living space can keep airways moist and reduce congestion.
- **Rest**: Your body heals best when it's well-rested. Aim for quality sleep to support your recovery process.

Finding natural remedies for common ailments like chest congestion can empower you to take charge of your health. This herbal infusion of eucalyptus and thyme provides a gentle, effective way to alleviate symptoms while nourishing your body.

5. Herbal Healing Recipe for Acne: Nature's Approach to Clear Skin

Acne is a common skin condition that affects millions of people worldwide, transcending age, gender, and even lifestyle. While conventional treatments can be effective, many individuals seek natural remedies to minimize side effects and promote overall skin health. The beauty of herbal healing lies in its natural ingredients that possess anti-inflammatory, antibacterial, and soothing properties.

Understanding Acne and Its Causes

Before we dive into the herbal recipe, it's vital to understand what acne is. Acne occurs when hair follicles become clogged with oil (sebum) and dead skin cells. This blockage can lead to inflammation and bacterial growth, often resulting in pimples, blackheads, and cysts. Common causes of acne include:

- Hormonal changes (especially during puberty, menstruation, and pregnancy)
- Excess oil production
- Bacteria on the skin
- Stress
- Diet (high in sugar and processed foods)
- Certain medications

While numerous treatment options are available, it's crucial to find an approach that aligns with your body's needs and minimizes potential side effects. Herbal remedies may offer a gentler solution.

Herbal Acne Clearing Recipe

Below is an easy-to-make herbal remedy that you can prepare at home. This recipe combines several potent herbs known for their acne-fighting properties.

Ingredients:

- **1 tablespoon dried chamomile flowers**: Chamomile is renowned for its anti-inflammatory properties, helping to reduce redness and irritation associated with acne.
- **1 tablespoon dried calendula petals**: Calendula possesses antibacterial and anti-inflammatory properties, which can help soothe the skin and promote healing.
- **1 tablespoon dried lavender flowers**: Lavender has antimicrobial properties and helps balance oil production while calming the skin.
- **1 cup distilled water**: Softens the herbs for effective extraction and is clean for topical use.
- **1 tablespoon raw honey (optional)**: Honey has natural antibacterial properties and acts as a humectant, keeping your skin moisturized.

Instructions:

1. **Herbal Infusion**: In a small saucepan, combine the chamomile, calendula, and lavender with the distilled water. Bring the mixture to a gentle simmer over low heat. Let it simmer for about 10 minutes to allow the beneficial properties of the herbs to infuse into the water.
2. **Strain**: After 10 minutes, remove the saucepan from heat. Strain the liquid into a clean bowl or glass jar, discarding the herbal solids.
3. **Add Honey**: If you choose to use honey, stir it into the warm herbal infusion until fully dissolved. This step is optional but can enhance the healing properties of the blend.
4. **Cool Down**: Allow the mixture to cool to room temperature before use.

Application:

- **Toner**: Once cooled, you can use this herbal infusion as a toner. Apply it to a clean face using a cotton ball or pad, focusing on areas with acne. Leave it on for about 10-15 minutes, then rinse off with cool water.
- **Spot Treatment**: For concentrated treatment, soak a clean cotton swab in the herbal solution and apply it directly to the affected areas. Allow it to sit for a few hours or overnight for maximum effect.

- **Storage**: Store any unused herbal infusion in the refrigerator for up to one week. Always give it a quick shake or stir before using, as the ingredients may settle.

Additional Tips for Clear Skin

While this herbal remedy can be beneficial for acne, combining it with a holistic approach will yield better results:

- **Stay Hydrated**: Drink plenty of water to keep your skin hydrated from the inside out.
- **Balanced Diet**: Incorporate a diet rich in whole foods, fruits, vegetables, and healthy fats while minimizing sugar and dairy intake.
- **Skin Care Routine**: Establish a consistent skincare regimen that includes gentle cleansing, exfoliating, and moisturizing to keep your skin balanced.
- **Consult a Professional**: If your acne persists or worsens, consider consulting a dermatologist or herbalist for tailored advice and treatment options.

Herbal remedies offer a gentle and natural approach to managing acne. This simple recipe harnesses the power of chamomile, calendula, and lavender to provide relief from inflammation and promote skin healing. Remember that everyone's skin is unique, and what works for one person may not work for another. Always perform a patch test to ensure you don't have any adverse reactions to the herbal ingredients. By nurturing your skin with nature's goodness, you can embark on a journey toward clearer, healthier skin. Happy healing!

6. Herbal Healing Recipe for Kidney Stones: Embracing Nature's Remedies

Kidney stones are not just a health nuisance; they can be incredibly painful and often lead to significant lifestyle changes while we seek ways to manage their formation. If you're looking for natural approaches to alleviate discomfort and potentially minimize the risk of future stones, herbal remedies may offer a supportive role in your journey toward better kidney health.

Understanding Kidney Stones

Before we dive into our herbal remedy, let's take a moment to understand what kidney stones are. These are Hard mineral and salt deposits that form inside your kidneys, often resulting from high levels of certain substances in your urine. Factors like dehydration, poor diet, obesity, and certain medical conditions can increase your risk. Symptoms can include severe pain in the side and back, blood in the urine, and nausea.

Herbal Healing Recipe: Kidney Stone Tea

Ingredients

1. **Hydrangea Root** (4 tablespoons) - Known for its diuretic properties, hydrangea root

can help flush out kidney stones and alleviate discomfort.

2. **Uva Ursi (Bearberry Leaf)** (2 tablespoons) - This herb has antibacterial properties and is traditionally used to support urinary tract health while promoting stone expulsion.
3. **Dandelion Root** (2 tablespoons) - Dandelion supports liver function and helps detoxify the body, which can be beneficial for kidney health.
4. **Nettle Leaf** (2 tablespoons) - This herb is rich in nutrients and serves as a natural diuretic, promoting urine flow and supporting the kidneys.
5. **Water** (8 cups) - Essential for brewing our herbal tea and promoting hydration.

Preparation

1. **Combine the Herbs**: In a large pot, combine the hydrangea root, uva ursi leaves, dandelion root, and nettle leaves.
2. **Boil Water**: Bring 8 cups of water to a rolling boil.
3. **Steep the Herbs**: Pour the boiling water over the herbs. Cover the pot and let the mixture steep for about 30 minutes to 1 hour. This allows the nutrients and beneficial compounds of the herbs to infuse into the water.
4. **Strain the Tea**: After steeping, strain the tea into a clean container. Discard the herb remains.
5. **Drink Daily**: Drink up to 2-3 cups of this herbal tea daily, preferably throughout

the day. You can also add honey or lemon for extra flavor, but be cautious with sugar if you are managing your diet closely.

Tips for Success

- **Stay Hydrated**: In addition to your herbal tea, ensure you are drinking plenty of other fluids to support your body in flushing out stones.
- **Adjust Your Diet**: Incorporate foods rich in fiber, potassium, and magnesium while reducing sodium and oxalate-rich foods such as spinach and nuts.
- **Consult a Healthcare Professional**: If you have a history of kidney stones or any ongoing health issues, consult with a healthcare provider before starting any herbal remedies.

While herbal remedies are a natural approach to managing kidney stones, they should not replace medical advice or treatment. Dandelion, uva ursi, hydrangea, and nettle are ancient allies in supporting kidney health and might provide relief, but individual responses can vary. Use this recipe as a nourishing support in your wellness journey, alongside a balanced diet and proper hydration. Remember, your kidneys do an incredible job filtering waste, so treat them kindly with nature's remedies!

Stay healthy, and may your journey toward wellness be filled with herbs and good intentions!

7. Natural Relief: An Herbal Healing Recipe for Constipation

Constipation is a common digestive issue that affects people of all ages. It can lead to discomfort, bloating, and an overall sense of sluggishness. While there are many over-the-counter remedies available, you might find solace in the healing properties of herbs. Below, we'll explore a simple and effective herbal healing recipe designed to alleviate constipation and promote regularity.

Understanding Constipation

Before diving into the herbal remedy, it's important to understand what constipation is. Generally defined as having fewer than three bowel movements per week, constipation can also involve hard stools and straining during bowel movements. Factors contributing to constipation can include inadequate fiber intake, dehydration, lack of physical activity, and certain medications.

Why Choose Herbs?

Herbal remedies can provide a natural solution to discomfort without the potential side effects associated with pharmaceuticals. Many herbs possess gentle laxative effects, support digestive health, and encourage regular elimination.

Herbal Healing Recipe: Soothing Digestive Tea

Ingredients:

1. **Dandelion Root** (1 teaspoon, dried)
2. **Senna Leaf** (1 teaspoon, dried)
3. **Fennel Seeds** (1 teaspoon, whole)
4. **Ginger Root** (1 teaspoon, grated or dried)
5. **Peppermint Leaf** (1 teaspoon, dried)
6. **Honey** (optional, for sweetness)
7. **Water** (2 cups)

Instructions:

1. **Prepare the Ingredients**: Gather all your dried herbs. If you're using fresh ginger, peel and grate it.
2. **Boil the Water**: In a medium-sized pot, bring 2 cups of water to a gentle boil.
3. **Combine the Herbs**: Once the water is boiling, remove it from heat and add the dandelion root, senna leaf, fennel seeds, ginger, and peppermint.
4. **Steep**: Cover the pot and allow the herbs to steep for about 10-15 minutes. This will ensure that the beneficial compounds in the herbs are released into the water.
5. **Strain and Serve**: After steeping, strain the tea into a cup. Add honey to taste if you prefer a little sweetness.
6. **Enjoy**: Drink the herbal tea while it's warm. For best results, enjoy this tea in the evening before bedtime or in the morning for a gentle morning boost.

How It Works:

- **Dandelion Root**: Known for its detoxifying properties, dandelion root helps stimulate bile production, which aids digestion.
- **Senna Leaf**: This herb is a natural laxative that promotes bowel movements by stimulating the muscles of the intestines.
- **Fennel Seeds**: Rich in fiber, fennel can help improve digestion and reduce bloating.
- **Ginger Root**: Ginger is famous for its ability to soothe the stomach and promote overall digestive health.
- **Peppermint Leaf**: This refreshing herb aids digestion by relaxing the muscles of the gastrointestinal tract.

Precautions:

1. **Dosage**: Senna should not be taken in excess or for extended periods, as it can lead to dependency or diminished bowel function. Use this tea as a temporary remedy.
2. **Consult a Professional**: If you experience chronic constipation or have underlying health issues, it's best to consult a healthcare professional before trying herbal remedies.
3. **Individual Reactions**: Everyone's body responds differently to herbs. Monitor how you feel after consuming this tea.

Complementary Lifestyle Tips

In addition to this herbal tea, consider the following tips for promoting digestive health and preventing constipation:

- **Stay Hydrated**: Drink plenty of water throughout the day.
- **Increase Fiber Intake**: Include more fiber-rich foods in your diet, such as fruits, vegetables, whole grains, and legumes.
- **Exercise Regularly**: Physical activity can stimulate digestion, making it easier for your body to process food.
- **Establish a Routine**: Try to set a regular time each day to use the restroom, allowing your body to develop a natural rhythm.

Constipation can be uncomfortable, but nature offers powerful solutions. This herbal healing recipe for constipation not only soothes digestive distress but also connects you to the healing properties of plants. Remember, while this tea can be a helpful remedy, maintaining a balanced lifestyle with proper hydration, nutrition, and exercise is key to long-term digestive health. Always listen to your body, and consult with a healthcare provider when necessary. Embrace the power of nature and take your first step towards a healthier digestive system today!

8. Herbal Healing Recipe for Flu: Boost Your Immunity Naturally

As the cold and flu season rolls around, many of us look for ways to strengthen our immune system and ease the symptoms that come with viral infections. While conventional medicine has its place, turning to nature's pharmacy can offer gentle yet effective remedies. In this section, we'll explore an herbal healing recipe that not only soothes flu symptoms but also helps bolster your body's defenses.

The Power of Herbs in Flu Recovery

Herbs have been used for centuries in traditional medicine systems around the world. Many of these plants offer antiviral, anti-inflammatory, and immune-boosting properties. When it comes to flu symptoms, certain herbs can help relieve congestion, soothe sore throats, reduce fever, and promote better overall health.

Key Ingredients for Our Herbal Flu Remedy

1. **Elderberry**: Known for its potent antiviral properties, elderberry extract can help reduce the severity and duration of flu symptoms. It's packed with antioxidants and can promote overall immune function.

2. **Ginger**: This warming herb acts as a natural anti-inflammatory and can help alleviate sore throats and make breathing easier. Ginger also works as a digestive aid, which is helpful if flu symptoms include nausea.
3. **Garlic**: This powerful bulb has been shown to enhance immune function and has antiviral properties. Garlic can be beneficial for the respiratory system and is known for its detoxifying effects.
4. **Chamomile**: Often used as a calming tea, chamomile can reduce inflammation and provide relief for upset stomachs. Its gentle sedative properties can help with rest, which is crucial for recovery.
5. **Honey**: While not an herb, honey is an essential addition for its soothing properties and its ability to coat the throat. Raw honey also has antimicrobial qualities that can further bolster recovery.

Herbal Flu Tea Recipe

Here's a delicious and soothing tea recipe that brings together the aforementioned ingredients to help combat flu symptoms:

Ingredients:

- 1 tablespoon dried elderberries (or 1/4 cup fresh elderberries)
- 1 tablespoon grated fresh ginger (or 1 teaspoon dried ginger)
- 2 cloves of garlic, crushed

- 1 tablespoon dried chamomile flowers
- 2 cups water
- 1 to 2 tablespoons raw honey (to taste)
- Optional: juice of half a lemon for added vitamin C

Instructions:

1. **Prepare the Elderberry**: If using fresh elderberries, make sure to wash them thoroughly and remove any stems. Dried elderberries can be used directly.
2. **Boil the Herbs**: In a saucepan, combine the elderberries, ginger, garlic, and chamomile with 2 cups of water. Bring the mixture to a boil over medium heat.
3. **Simmer**: Once it reaches a boil, reduce the heat and let it simmer for about 15-20 minutes. This allows the flavors and beneficial properties to infuse into the water.
4. **Strain**: After simmering, remove the pot from heat and strain the mixture into a teapot or large mug. This will remove the solid ingredients, leaving you with a soothing tea.
5. **Sweeten and Serve**: While the tea is still warm, stir in the raw honey and lemon juice if desired. Adjust the sweetness to your taste.
6. **Enjoy**: Sip the tea slowly, allowing it to soothe your throat and warm your body. This remedy can be consumed 2-3 times a day while you're feeling under the weather.

Additional Tips for Flu Prevention

- **Stay Hydrated**: Drink plenty of fluids to help your body flush out toxins.
- **Rest**: Your body needs rest to recover; don't underestimate the power of sleep.
- **Healthy Diet**: Load up on nutrient-dense foods, including fruits and vegetables, which support immune health.
- **Wash Your Hands**: Good hygiene can help prevent the spread of germs and keep you healthier during flu season.

When to Seek Medical Help

While herbal remedies can be effective for mild flu symptoms, it's essential to listen to your body. If you experience high fever, difficulty breathing, or any severe symptoms, make sure to consult a healthcare professional right away.

Herbal healing offers a holistic approach to managing flu symptoms while supporting your immune system. Integrating this herbal tea recipe into your toolkit can help you navigate the flu season with greater ease. Remember, self-care is essential, especially during illness — so take the time to rest and nourish your body. Cheers to health and wellness!

9. Herbal Healing for Irritable Bowel Syndrome: A Soothing Recipe

Irritable Bowel Syndrome (IBS) affects millions of people worldwide, bringing discomfort and disruption to everyday life. While medical advice and interventions are crucial, many individuals find relief in natural remedies, especially those derived from herbs. If you're looking to soothe your digestive woes with herbal healing, this information here presents a simple, yet powerful herbal remedy designed to alleviate the symptoms of IBS.

Understanding Irritable Bowel Syndrome

IBS is a chronic functional gastrointestinal disorder characterized by symptoms such as abdominal pain, bloating, gas, and irregular bowel habits (diarrhea, constipation, or both). While the exact cause of IBS remains elusive, triggers can include stress, dietary choices, and hormonal changes.

Herbal remedies may serve as a complementary approach to managing symptoms, helping to calm the gut, reduce inflammation, and promote digestive health.

A Herbal Recipe for IBS Relief: Soothing Digestive Tea

One of the simplest and most effective ways to harness the power of herbs is through tea. This soothing digestive tea combines well-known herbs that have been traditionally used to ease digestive discomfort, calm the gut, and promote regularity.

Ingredients

- **1 teaspoon peppermint leaves**: Known for its antispasmodic properties, peppermint can help relax the muscles of the gastrointestinal tract. It's also effective in alleviating bloating and discomfort.
- **1 teaspoon ginger root (grated or dried)**: Ginger has long been used to combat nausea and aid digestion. Its anti-inflammatory properties can help soothe an irritated gut.
- **1 teaspoon chamomile flowers**: Chamomile is an excellent herb for relaxation and calming abdominal distress. It has anti-inflammatory and anti-anxiety effects that can be beneficial for those with IBS.
- **1 teaspoon fennel seeds**: Fennel helps to relieve bloating and gas while promoting healthy digestion. Its carminative properties can significantly ease abdominal discomfort.
- **2 cups of boiling water**

Instructions

1. **Combine the Herbs**: In a teapot or heatproof container, combine the

peppermint leaves, ginger root, chamomile
flowers, and fennel seeds.
2. **Pour the Water**: Carefully pour the boiling
water over the herbs.
3. **Steep**: Cover the container and let the
herbal mixture steep for 10-15 minutes.
This allows the flavors and beneficial
properties of the herbs to infuse into the
water.
4. **Strain and Serve**: After steeping, strain the
tea into a cup. You can add a teaspoon of
honey or a slice of lemon for added flavor—
both can boost digestive health.
5. **Enjoy**: Sip your herbal tea slowly,
preferably after meals or whenever you feel
gastrointestinal discomfort.

Tips for Use

- **Frequency**: Drink this soothing tea 1-2
  times daily, especially during flare-ups or
  when consuming trigger foods.
- **Listen to Your Body**: As with any herbal
  remedy, it's essential to pay attention to
  how your body responds. Adjust the
  ingredients or frequency according to your
  comfort and tolerance.
- **Stay Hydrated**: Complement this tea with
  plenty of water throughout the day to
  support overall digestive health.

Final Thoughts

While this herbal tea can be a supportive remedy
for managing IBS symptoms, always consult with

a healthcare professional before incorporating new treatments into your routine, especially if you are taking medications or have underlying health conditions. Managing IBS often requires a multifaceted approach, including dietary changes, stress management, and lifestyle modifications. Embracing herbal healing is a wonderful addition to this journey, offering a natural way to find relief and improve your overall well-being.

Remember, nature offers a wealth of remedies— take a moment to savor this soothing herbal tea and help restore balance to your digestive system. Happy sipping!

10. Herbal Healing for Anxiety: A Soothing Recipe to Calm Your Mind

In today's fast-paced world, anxiety has become a common experience for many people. With the pressures of work, family, and everyday life, finding peace and calm can often feel like an uphill battle. While coping mechanisms vary from person to person, many are turning to herbal remedies for relief. Not only do herbs nurture the body, but they can also soothe the mind and help restore balance.

The Power of Herbs

Herbs have been used for centuries in traditional medicine across various cultures. Many have calming properties that can help reduce symptoms of anxiety. Common herbs associated with calming effects include:

- **Chamomile**: Known for its soothing effects, chamomile can help reduce tension and promote sleep.
- **Lavender**: This fragrant herb is often used for its calming scent, which can help alleviate stress and anxiety.
- **Lemon Balm**: Traditionally used to ease anxiety, lemon balm can enhance mood and improve sleep quality.

- **Passionflower**: Often used to treat anxiety and insomnia, passionflower can help you relax without the groggy aftereffects of some medications.

Herbal Healing Recipe: Calming Herbal Tea Blend

Creating your own herbal tea is a wonderful way to incorporate these herbs into your daily routine. Below is a simple recipe that can help ease anxiety and promote a sense of calm.

Ingredients:

- 1 tablespoon dried chamomile flowers
- 1 tablespoon dried lavender flowers
- 1 tablespoon dried lemon balm leaves
- 1 tablespoon dried passionflower
- 4 cups of filtered water
- Honey or lemon (optional, for taste)

Instructions:

1. **Combine the Herbs**: In a small bowl, mix the dried chamomile, lavender, lemon balm, and passionflower together. This blend can be stored in an airtight container for future use.
2. **Boil the Water**: In a saucepan, bring 4 cups of filtered water to a boil.
3. **Steep the Herbs**: Once the water is boiling, remove it from the heat and add the herbal blend. Cover the saucepan and let it steep for about 10 minutes. This allows the herbs to release their beneficial compounds.

4. **Strain and Serve**: After steeping, strain the tea into your favorite mug. If desired, add honey or lemon for a touch of sweetness or acidity.
5. **Enjoy Mindfully**: Sit down in a quiet space, sip your tea slowly, and take a moment to breathe deeply. Engaging in a mindful practice while enjoying your tea can enhance its calming effects.

Additional Tips for Anxiety Management

While this herbal tea can provide relief, consider incorporating these healthy practices into your routine for holistic well-being:

- **Mindfulness and Meditation**: Practicing mindfulness or meditation for even just a few minutes a day can significantly reduce anxiety levels.
- **Regular Exercise**: Physical activity releases endorphins, which can help elevate your mood and reduce stress.
- **Adequate Sleep**: Aim for 7-9 hours of quality sleep each night to help regulate emotions and improve overall mental health.
- **Healthy Diet**: Incorporate a balanced diet rich in fruits, vegetables, whole grains, and healthy fats to fuel your body and mind.

Final Word

Anxiety can feel overwhelming, but nature has provided us with powerful tools to help manage it.

This calming herbal tea blend is a delightful way to incorporate soothing herbs into your daily routine. As you sip and savor each moment, remember to listen to your body and mind. While herbal remedies can offer significant support, don't hesitate to reach out to a healthcare professional if your anxiety persists or worsens. Together with your herbal allies and a holistic lifestyle approach, you can find your path to inner peace. Enjoy your brewing journey!

11. Herbal Healing Recipe for Lower Back Pain: Nature's Remedy

Lower back pain is a common ailment that affects millions of people around the world, often making everyday activities difficult and uncomfortable. While there are countless medications and therapies available, many individuals are turning to nature for relief. Herbal remedies can offer soothing effects that can help alleviate pain and promote healing. Here, we will explore an herbal healing recipe designed to ease lower back pain, combining the effectiveness of specific herbs known for their anti-inflammatory and analgesic properties.

Understanding Lower Back Pain

Before diving into our herbal remedy, it's important to understand what causes lower back pain. It can result from various factors, including muscle or ligament strain, herniated discs, arthritis, and even stress. Chronic pain can be debilitating, but natural remedies can provide a supportive approach to managing discomfort.

The Power of Herbs

Herbs have been used for centuries in traditional medicine to heal various ailments, including back pain. Here are some key players in our herbal healing recipe:

1. **Turmeric:** Known for its anti-inflammatory properties, turmeric contains curcumin, which can help reduce swelling and pain. It's often used to treat conditions like arthritis.
2. **Ginger:** With its natural analgesic effects, ginger can help reduce inflammation and promote circulation, easing muscle tension and pain.
3. **Comfrey:** Often used topically, comfrey can promote healing in the muscles and soft tissues due to its ability to stimulate cell regeneration. However, it should be used with caution, as it should not be ingested over the long term.
4. **Peppermint:** Known for its cooling effect, peppermint can help relieve pain and reduce muscle spasms.
5. **Cayenne Pepper:** Containing capsaicin, cayenne pepper can reduce pain signals sent to the brain, providing temporary relief from discomfort.

Herbal Healing Recipe: Back Pain Relief Salve

Ingredients

- 1 cup coconut oil (or olive oil)
- 2 tablespoons dried turmeric root (or 1 tablespoon fresh turmeric)
- 1 tablespoon dried ginger root (or 1 tablespoon fresh ginger)
- 1 tablespoon dried comfrey leaves (ensure safe usage guidelines)
- 1 tablespoon dried peppermint leaves

- 1 teaspoon cayenne pepper (adjust for sensitivity)
- 1 ounce beeswax (if you prefer a firmer salve)
- Optional: Essential oils like eucalyptus or lavender for added healing properties

Instructions

1. **Infuse the Oils:**
   - In a double boiler, combine the coconut oil and dried herbs (turmeric, ginger, comfrey, peppermint, and cayenne).
   - Heat on low for about 1-2 hours, allowing the oils to absorb the beneficial properties of the herbs. Stir occasionally and be careful not to overheat.
2. **Strain the Mixture:**
   - Once the infusion is complete, strain the oil through a fine mesh strainer or cheesecloth into a clean bowl to remove the solid herbs.
3. **Add Beeswax:**
   - Return the infused oil to the double boiler and add beeswax if you want to create a more solid salve. Use approximately 1 ounce for a firmer texture.
   - Heat until the beeswax is fully melted and combined.
4. **Cool and Add Essential Oils:**
   - Remove from heat and let it cool slightly before adding a few drops of

your chosen essential oils for added fragrance and healing properties.

5. **Pour into Containers:**
   - Once the mixture is well combined, carefully pour it into small jars or tins and allow it to cool completely.
6. **Storage:**
   - Store your herbal salve in a cool, dark place. It should last several months if kept clean and properly sealed.

How to Use the Salve

To use your herbal salve, simply apply a small amount to the affected area of your lower back and massage it gently into the skin. The warmth from your hands will help activate the herbs' properties, allowing for deeper penetration. For best results, use it 2-3 times daily or as needed.

Important Notes

- **Consultation:** Always consult with a healthcare provider before starting any new treatment, especially if you have pre-existing conditions or are pregnant or nursing.
- **Patch Test:** Perform a patch test to ensure you don't have an allergic reaction to any ingredients.
- **Limitations:** This salve is for external use only; do not ingest the comfrey salve as it can be toxic in large amounts when consumed.

Lower back pain can be a nuisance, but nature provides many remedies that can help soothe and support our bodies. This herbal healing salve combines the power of turmeric, ginger, comfrey, peppermint, and cayenne pepper to create a natural, effective treatment for relief. Always listen to your body and consult healthcare professionals if your pain persists.

Embrace the natural healing power of herbs; your back will thank you!

12. Herbal Healing Recipe for Acid Reflux: Finding Relief Naturally

Acid reflux, also known as gastro esophageal reflux disease (GERD), can be a frustrating and uncomfortable condition. Characterized by a burning sensation in the chest, a bitter taste in the mouth, and other digestive disturbances, many individuals find themselves seeking both lifestyle changes and remedies to alleviate their symptoms. While over-the-counter medications are widely available, many are turning towards herbal remedies for a more holistic approach to healing.

Understanding Acid Reflux

Before diving into our herbal remedy, it's important to understand what acid reflux is. When the lower esophageal sphincter (LES) doesn't close properly, stomach acid can flow back into the esophagus, causing irritation. Factors contributing to acid reflux can include diet, obesity, smoking, and pregnancy. A healthier lifestyle, combined with natural remedies, can play a key role in alleviating symptoms.

Herbal Ingredients That Help

The following herbs are known for their soothing properties and can help combat the symptoms of acid reflux:

1. **Ginger**: Renowned for its anti-inflammatory properties, ginger can help reduce nausea and promote digestion.
2. **Chamomile**: This calming herb is traditionally used to promote relaxation and counter irritation in the digestive tract.
3. **Slippery Elm**: This herb contains mucilage, a gel-like substance that coats the stomach and esophagus, providing a protective barrier against acid.
4. **Licorice Root**: Used for centuries to soothe digestive discomfort, it helps to rebuild the stomach's protective mucous lining.
5. **Fennel**: This aromatic herb aids digestion and can help reduce bloating and gas, often accompanying acid reflux.

Herbal Healing Recipe: Soothing Chamomile-Ginger Tea

This comforting tea blends the anti-inflammatory and digestive benefits of several herbs, creating a calming remedy for acid reflux. It's easy to make and can be enjoyed daily.

Ingredients:

- 1 cup of water
- 1 teaspoon dried chamomile flowers (or 1 chamomile tea bag)
- 1 teaspoon fresh ginger, grated (or 1/2 teaspoon dried ginger)
- 1 teaspoon slippery elm powder (optional for extra soothing effect)
- 1 teaspoon honey (optional, for sweetness)

- A slice of lemon (optional, use sparingly as citrus can trigger reflux in some people)

Instructions:

1. **Boil the Water**: In a small saucepan, bring the cup of water to a boil.
2. **Add the Herbs**: Once boiling, remove from heat and add the chamomile flowers and grated ginger. If using slippery elm, add it now.
3. **Steep**: Cover the pot and let the mixture steep for about 10 minutes. This allows the beneficial compounds to permeate the water, creating a flavorful and effective tea.
4. **Strain and Serve**: After steeping, strain the tea into a cup. If desired, add honey for sweetness and a slice of lemon for extra flavor. Remember to use lemon cautiously; for some, it can aggravate symptoms.
5. **Enjoy**: Sip your tea slowly, ideally after meals or when you feel an acid reflux flare-up coming on. The warmth of the tea will provide soothing relief while the herbs work their magic.

Additional Tips for Managing Acid Reflux

In addition to this herbal remedy, here are some lifestyle changes you can make to further manage acid reflux:

- **Eat smaller meals**: Large meals can put pressure on the LES, leading to reflux. Opt for smaller, more frequent meals.

- **Avoid trigger foods**: Common culprits include spicy foods, fatty foods, mint, chocolate, caffeine, and acidic foods.
- **Stay upright after eating**: Try to avoid lying down for at least 3 hours after meals.
- **Maintain a healthy weight**: Excess weight can put more pressure on your abdomen and LES.
- **Practice stress-reducing techniques**: Stress management through yoga, meditation, and deep-breathing exercises can positively impact digestion.

Herbal remedies can be a valuable part of managing acid reflux symptoms, offering gentle yet effective relief without the side effects of conventional medications. By incorporating soothing herbal teas like our chamomile-ginger blend into your routine, alongside other healthy lifestyle changes, you can regain comfort and wellbeing. Remember, it's always best to consult with a healthcare professional before starting any new treatment, especially if you have underlying health conditions or are taking medications.

Here's to your health—naturally!

13. Herbal Healing for Psoriasis: A Natural Recipe to Soothe Your Skin

Psoriasis is a chronic autoimmune condition characterized by red, inflamed patches of skin covered with silvery scales. While conventional treatments can be effective, many individuals are seeking alternative methods, including herbal remedies, to manage symptoms and promote skin health.

Why Choose Herbal Remedies?

Herbal remedies have been used for centuries to treat various skin conditions, including psoriasis. Unlike conventional medications, which may come with side effects, herbal treatments can offer a more holistic approach, supporting the body's natural healing processes. Key benefits of using herbal remedies for psoriasis include:

- **Natural Ingredients**: Many herbs are anti-inflammatory, antiseptic, and rich in antioxidants, making them suitable for soothing irritated skin.
- **Fewer Side Effects**: Herbal remedies often have fewer side effects compared to conventional medications.
- **Personal Empowerment**: Using herbal remedies can empower individuals to take

control of their healing process and explore natural options.

Key Ingredients for Our Herbal Healing Recipe

For our herbal healing recipe, we're focusing on ingredients known for their skin-soothing properties:

1. **Aloe Vera**: This succulent plant is renowned for its ability to hydrate and soothe the skin, thanks to its anti-inflammatory and healing properties.
2. **Calendula**: Known for its anti-inflammatory and antimicrobial benefits, calendula helps to heal wounds and reduce redness.
3. **Chamomile**: Chamomile possesses calming effects and can help reduce inflammation, irritation, and itching associated with psoriasis.
4. **Neem Oil**: Neem has antifungal, antibacterial, and anti-inflammatory properties, making it an excellent choice for treating skin conditions.
5. **Coconut Oil**: With its moisturizing properties, coconut oil helps to hydrate the skin and reduce dryness and scaling.

Herbal Healing Recipe for Psoriasis

Soothing Herbal Salve

Ingredients:

- 1/4 cup dried aloe vera gel (or fresh, if available)
- 1/4 cup dried calendula flowers
- 1/4 cup dried chamomile flowers
- 1/4 cup coconut oil
- 1 tablespoon neem oil
- 1 tablespoon beeswax (optional, for a thicker consistency)
- 10-15 drops of lavender essential oil (optional for fragrance)

Instructions:

1. **Prepare the Herbal Infusion**:
   - In a saucepan, combine the calendula flowers and chamomile flowers with coconut oil.
   - Gently heat the mixture over low heat for about 20-30 minutes, ensuring it doesn't boil. This process allows the oil to absorb the beneficial properties of the herbs.
2. **Strain the Mixture**:
   - After infusing, strain the oil through a fine mesh strainer or cheesecloth to remove the herb particles. You should have a beautifully golden oil.
3. **Combine with Aloe Vera**:
   - In a clean, dry bowl, mix the infused oil with the aloe vera gel and neem oil. Stir until well combined.
4. **Add Beeswax (Optional)**:
   - If you prefer a thicker salve, melt the beeswax in the saucepan over low

heat and then combine it with the oil mixture. Stir until fully incorporated.
5. **Essential Oils**:
    - If using, add lavender essential oil for fragrance and additional calming properties. Stir well.
6. **Cool and Store**:
    - Pour the mixture into a clean glass jar or container. Allow it to cool completely before sealing the lid. Store your salve in a cool, dry place for up to six months.

How to Use the Salve

- Apply the salve directly to the affected areas of the skin once or twice daily, especially after bathing.
- Gently massage the salve into the skin, allowing your body to absorb the healing benefits of the herbs.
- For optimal results, combine this topical treatment with a holistic approach to manage psoriasis, including a balanced diet and stress management techniques.

Final Thoughts

While this herbal healing recipe can provide relief for psoriasis symptoms, it's essential to consult with a healthcare professional before starting any new treatment, especially if you're taking medication or dealing with severe symptoms. Remember, psoriasis is a complex condition, and what works for one person may not work for another. Choosing natural remedies can be a beautiful journey toward healing. By understanding the power of herbs, you can find soothing relief while nurturing your skin with gentle, effective care.

Happy healing!

14. Herbal Healing for Cystic Fibrosis: A Natural Approach to Wellness

Cystic Fibrosis (CF) is a genetic condition that primarily affects the lungs and digestive system, leading to thick mucus buildup. This can cause breathing difficulties and digestive issues, necessitating ongoing medical treatment. While conventional medicine plays a crucial role in managing CF, many individuals and families are turning to holistic approaches to augment their care. One such avenue is the use of herbal remedies to support lung health and overall well-being.

Understanding Cystic Fibrosis

Before diving into herbal remedies, it's imperative to recognize that cystic fibrosis is a serious condition that requires a comprehensive care plan designed by healthcare professionals. Herbal remedies can complement traditional treatments but should not replace them. If you or a loved one is considering herbal therapies, always consult with a qualified healthcare provider to ensure safety and appropriateness.

The Role of Herbs in Supporting Lung Health

Herbs have been used for centuries in traditional medicine systems for their healing properties.

Certain herbs can help with respiratory function, reduce inflammation, and improve overall health. Here are a few notable herbs that may offer support for individuals with CF:

1. **Mullein (Verbascum thapsus)**: Known for its ability to soothe the respiratory system, mullein acts as an expectorant, helping to expel mucus from the lungs.
2. **Thyme (Thymus vulgaris)**: This herb has antiseptic and anti-inflammatory properties that can help clear up respiratory infections. It also acts as a bronchial dilator, making it easier to breathe.
3. **Ginger (Zingiber officinale)**: Ginger has potent anti-inflammatory properties and can help ease digestive difficulties often associated with CF, as well as improve respiratory health.
4. **Licorice Root (Glycyrrhiza glabra)**: This herb has soothing properties that help reduce irritation in the throat and respiratory tract, making it easier to manage coughs.
5. **Osha Root (Ligusticum porteri)**: Traditionally used by Native Americans, Osha Root is known for its ability to support lung health and relieve respiratory distress.

An Herbal Healing Recipe for Cystic Fibrosis

Here's a simple herbal infusion recipe using a combination of the above herbs. This tea can act as a supportive remedy to promote lung health and alleviate some symptoms, but remember, it's not a replacement for prescribed treatments.

Ingredients:

- 1 teaspoon dried mullein leaves
- 1 teaspoon dried thyme leaves
- 1 teaspoon dried ginger root (or 1 teaspoon fresh grated ginger)
- 1 teaspoon dried licorice root (optional, especially for those with high blood pressure)
- 1 cup hot water
- Honey or lemon (optional, for taste)

Instructions:

1. **Prepare Your Herbs**: If using dried herbs, measure out the needed amounts. If you're using fresh ginger, grate it finely.
2. **Combine the Herbs**: In a heatproof container or teapot, combine all the dried herbs.
3. **Add Water**: Pour hot water (just below boiling) over the herbs.
4. **Steep**: Cover and let the mixture steep for about 10 to 15 minutes. This allows the beneficial properties of the herbs to infuse into the water.
5. **Strain**: After steeping, strain the herbs from the tea using a fine mesh strainer or tea infuser.
6. **Flavor (Optional)**: Add honey or lemon to taste if desired.
7. **Enjoy**: Sip the herbal infusion slowly, ideally 1 to 2 times per day.

Important Considerations

- **Consult with Your Healthcare Provider**: Always discuss with your doctor or a qualified herbalist before incorporating any new herbs into your routine, particularly for specific health conditions like CF.
- **Monitor for Allergies**: When trying any new herbal remedy, start with small amounts to test for any allergic reactions or side effects.
- **Lifestyle Factors**: Remember to also incorporate other beneficial practices such as a balanced diet, regular exercise (as tolerated), hydration, and stress management techniques into your wellness routine.

While cystic fibrosis remains a challenging condition requiring medical management, incorporating herbal remedies into a holistic approach can provide additional support and improve quality of life. By working closely with healthcare professionals and considering safe herbal options, individuals with CF can take proactive steps toward enhancing their health and well-being. The journey through Cystic Fibrosis can be complex, but with the right tools and support, it's possible to navigate it with resilience and hope.

15. An Herbal Healing Recipe for Liver Problems

The liver is one of the most vital organs in the human body, responsible for detoxification, metabolism, and nutrient synthesis. However, with the pressures of modern life—pollution, unhealthy diets, and excessive alcohol consumption—our livers often need a little extra care. Fortunately, nature provides us with a bounty of herbs that can support liver health.

The Importance of Liver Health

Before diving into our healing recipe, it's essential to understand why liver health is crucial. The liver performs functions such as:

- **Detoxification**: Filtering harmful substances from the blood, including toxins and drugs.
- **Metabolism**: Breaking down nutrients from food and converting them into usable forms.
- **Storage**: Storing vitamins, minerals, and energy sources for later use.
- **Bile Production**: Producing bile, which aids in digestion and absorption of fats.

Signs of liver distress can include fatigue, jaundice, digestive issues, and abdominal discomfort. If you are experiencing any of these symptoms, it is essential to consult a healthcare professional. This herbal recipe can be used as a complementary approach to support liver function.

Herbal Ingredients for Liver Health

The following herbs are known for their liver-supportive properties:

1. **Milk Thistle (Silybum marianum)**: Amino acids in milk thistle help repair liver cells and have powerful antioxidant properties, protecting the liver from damage.
2. **Dandelion Root (Taraxacum officinale)**: This common weed is a powerful liver tonic that stimulates bile production, aiding in digestion and detoxification.
3. **Turmeric (Curcuma longa)**: Curcumin, the active ingredient in turmeric, has potent anti-inflammatory properties and helps improve liver function.
4. **Licorice Root (Glycyrrhiza glabra)**: Known for its soothing properties, licorice root can help protect the liver against toxins and reduce inflammation.
5. **Peppermint (Mentha piperita)**: This refreshing herb aids digestion and promotes the effective functioning of the liver.

Herbal Liver Tonic Recipe

Ingredients

- 1 teaspoon dried milk thistle seeds

- 1 teaspoon dried dandelion root
- 1/2 teaspoon dried turmeric root (or 1/2 teaspoon of turmeric powder)
- 1/2 teaspoon dried licorice root
- 1 teaspoon dried peppermint leaves
- 4 cups water
- Honey or lemon (optional, for taste)

Instructions

1. **Combine the Herbs**: In a small glass or ceramic bowl, mix the dried milk thistle seeds, dandelion root, turmeric, licorice root, and peppermint leaves.
2. **Boil Water**: Bring 4 cups of water to a boil in a medium saucepan.
3. **Steep the Herbs**: Once the water reaches a full boil, remove it from heat. Add the combined herbs to the hot water. Cover and let steep for about 15-20 minutes. This allows the beneficial compounds to infuse into the water.
4. **Strain**: After steeping, strain the herbal mixture into a teapot or other container. Discard the leftover herbal debris.
5. **Add Flavor**: Optionally, sweeten your herbal tonic with honey or add a squeeze of lemon for added flavor and health benefits.
6. **Serve**: Drink your herbal liver tonic warm or chilled. Enjoy 1-2 cups daily to support liver health.

Final Thoughts

This herbal tonic is a gentle yet effective way to care for your liver naturally. However, remember that herbs can be potent, and it's crucial to consult with a healthcare provider before starting any new herbal regimen, particularly if you have existing health conditions or are taking medications. Beyond using herbal remedies, supporting liver health involves adopting a balanced diet rich in fruits, vegetables, and whole grains, staying hydrated, managing stress, and engaging in regular physical activity.

By incorporating this herbal healing recipe into your routine, you can take an encouraging step towards enhancing your liver health. Embrace the power of nature, and give your liver the love and support it deserves!

16. Herbal Healing: A Recipe for Thyroid Health

In today's fast-paced world, it's easy for us to overlook the importance of our thyroid, a small butterfly-shaped gland located in the neck that plays a crucial role in regulating metabolism, energy, and overall hormonal balance. Thyroid dysfunction, whether it be hypothyroidism (underactive thyroid) or hyperthyroidism (overactive thyroid), can lead to a myriad of health complications, including fatigue, weight changes, and mood disorders. While conventional medicine often provides effective treatments, many are turning to herbal remedies to complement their healing journey.

Let's explore an herbal recipe designed to support thyroid health, along with the benefits of the key ingredients.

Thyroid Support Herbal Infusion

Ingredients:

- **1 tablespoon dried Ashwagandha (Withania somnifera)**
- **1 tablespoon dried Nettle Leaf (Urtica dioica)**
- **1 tablespoon dried Bladderwrack (Fucus vesiculosus)**

- **1 tablespoon dried Licorice Root (Glycyrrhiza glabra)**
- **2 cups hot water**
- **Honey or lemon (optional, for taste)**

Instructions:

1. **Combine the Herbs**: In a teapot or a heatproof container, mix together the dried Ashwagandha, Nettle Leaf, Bladderwrack, and Licorice Root.
2. **Add Hot Water**: Pour the hot water over the herb mixture. Cover the teapot or container to trap the steam, which helps extract the beneficial compounds from the herbs.
3. **Steep the Mixture**: Allow the herbs to steep for about 10-15 minutes. This time will enable the water to absorb the beneficial properties of the herbs.
4. **Strain and Serve**: After steeping, strain the infusion into a cup. If desired, sweeten with honey or a splash of lemon for added flavor and health benefits.
5. **Enjoy**: Sip your herbal infusion 1-2 times daily. You can incorporate this into your morning routine or enjoy it as a relaxing afternoon beverage.

The Healing Power of the Ingredients

1. Ashwagandha: Known for its adaptogenic properties, Ashwagandha helps the body cope with stress, which can be particularly beneficial for thyroid health. Research has shown that it may improve thyroid hormone levels, making it a great addition for those with hypothyroidism.

2. Nettle Leaf: Rich in vitamins and minerals, including iron, magnesium, and vitamins A and C, nettle leaves are highly nutritious. Nettle can help improve energy levels and combat fatigue, which is particularly important for those suffering from low thyroid function.

3. Bladderwrack: This seaweed is a natural source of iodine, an essential nutrient for thyroid hormone production. Bladderwrack may help regulate thyroid function and support metabolic processes.

4. Licorice Root: Often used in traditional medicine for its soothing properties, Licorice root can help balance hormonal levels. It may enhance the efficacy of other herbs in this blend and provides a subtle sweetness to the infusion.

Important Considerations

While many people find relief and support from herbal remedies, it's essential to approach them with caution. Herbal treatments can interact with medications or conditions, so it's vital to consult with a healthcare provider before incorporating new herbs into your regimen, especially if you have a diagnosed thyroid condition or are currently on thyroid medication.

Additionally, lifestyle factors such as a balanced diet, regular exercise, and stress management techniques play a critical role in maintaining thyroid health. Herbs can be a wonderful ally in your wellness journey, but they are most effective when combined with a holistic approach. Taking care of your thyroid is crucial for maintaining overall health and well-being. This herbal infusion combines several powerful plants known for their supportive benefits to help nourish and balance the thyroid. Whether you're seeking to complement your existing treatment or embrace a herbal approach, this simple recipe can be an excellent addition. Always listen to your body and consult with health professionals as you explore the transformative potential of herbal healing.

Stay tuned for more herbal recipes and holistic health tips!

17. Herbal Healing Recipe for Cancer: Nature's Support in Times of Need

In the quest for holistic health, many individuals are turning to natural remedies to complement conventional cancer treatments. While it is crucial to emphasize that herbal remedies should never replace medical advice or treatments prescribed by healthcare professionals, some herbs have shown promise in supporting overall well-being and alleviating side effects associated with cancer. In this section, we'll explore a soothing herbal tea recipe that harnesses the healing properties of nature, along with some beneficial herbs linked to cancer support.

Understanding Herbal Support

Herbal medicine has been used for centuries to promote health and well-being. Certain herbs possess properties that may enhance the body's immune response, combat inflammation, and reduce stress—factors that can be vital during cancer treatment. However, it's essential to consult with a healthcare provider before integrating any herbal remedies into your routine, especially during cancer treatment, as some herbs can interact with conventional medications.

Healing Herbal Tea Recipe
Ingredients:

1. **Green Tea** (1 tsp) - Rich in antioxidants called catechins, green tea may help fight cancer cells and reduce tumor growth.
2. **Turmeric** (1 tsp) - Known for its active compound curcumin, turmeric has anti-inflammatory and antioxidant properties that may support the immune system.
3. **Ginger** (1 tsp, grated) - Ginger can help alleviate nausea and digestive issues, common side effects of chemotherapy, and has anti-inflammatory effects.
4. **Lemon Balm** (1 tsp) - This calming herb may help reduce anxiety and improve mood, contributing to emotional well-being.
5. **Honey** (to taste) - A natural sweetener with antibacterial properties that can soothe the throat and enhance the tea's flavor.
6. **Fresh Lemon Juice** (juice of half a lemon) - Rich in vitamin C, lemon can boost immunity and add a refreshing flavor.
7. **Water** (4 cups)

Instructions:

1. **Prepare the Base**: In a medium pot, bring 4 cups of water to a gentle boil.
2. **Add the Herbs**: Once the water reaches a boil, reduce the heat and add the green tea, turmeric, ginger, and lemon balm. Allow the mixture to simmer for about 10 minutes to extract the herbal benefits.
3. **Strain the Tea**: After simmering, strain the tea into a heatproof container to remove the solid herbs.

4. **Enhance Flavor**: Add the fresh lemon juice and honey to the strained tea, stirring until the honey is dissolved.
5. **Serve**: Enjoy the tea warm, or chill it in the refrigerator for a refreshing iced beverage later.

Additional Considerations

- **Frequency**: Enjoy this herbal tea daily or as needed, but listen to your body. If you experience any adverse reactions, discontinue use and consult your healthcare provider.
- **Customizable**: Feel free to experiment with other cancer-supporting herbs such as echinacea, ashwagandha, or milk thistle, depending on your individual needs and preferences.
- **Lifestyle Choices**: Incorporating this herbal tea into a balanced diet rich in fruits, vegetables, whole grains, and lean proteins can further enhance your overall health during treatment.

A Holistic Approach

While this herbal tea offers potential benefits, remember that cancer treatment is complex. Always prioritize discussions with healthcare professionals about your treatment plan and how herbal remedies can fit into your overall approach. Complementing medical treatment with supportive herbs can be a wonderful option, but they should be part of a well-rounded strategy focused on your health and wellness. Nature offers a wealth of healing options, and this herbal tea recipe is just one way to embrace the supportive properties of herbs during a challenging time. As you navigate cancer treatment, remember to remain hopeful, informed, and in close communication with your healthcare team. And remember to stay away from that sugar!

18. Herbal Healing Recipe for Diabetes: Embracing Nature's Remedies

As diabetes continues to affect millions worldwide, many are searching for natural and holistic approaches to managing this chronic condition. While it is essential to consult healthcare professionals before making any changes to medication or treatment plans, incorporating certain herbs into your diet can bolster your overall health and complement prescribed diabetes management strategies.

Understanding Diabetes and Herbal Remedies

Diabetes is characterized by elevated blood sugar levels due to problems with insulin production or utilization. There are two main types: Type 1 diabetes, where the body does not produce insulin, and Type 2 diabetes, which involves insulin resistance. Lifestyle changes, including diet and exercise, are vital in managing diabetes effectively.

Herbal remedies have long been used in traditional medicine systems to help regulate blood sugar levels, improve insulin sensitivity, and reduce complications related to diabetes. While herbs can be a beneficial addition to a diabetes-friendly lifestyle, it's crucial to remember that they should not replace conventional medical advice or treatment.

An Herbal Healing Recipe: Diabetic-Friendly Cinnamon Turmeric Tea

This simple yet powerful tea combines the anti-inflammatory and blood-sugar-lowering properties of cinnamon and turmeric, making it an excellent choice for those managing diabetes. Here's how to prepare it:

Ingredients:

- 1 cup of water
- ½ teaspoon of ground cinnamon (or 1 cinnamon stick)
- ½ teaspoon of ground turmeric (or 1-inch piece of fresh turmeric)
- 1 teaspoon of freshly squeezed lemon juice
- 1 teaspoon of honey (optional, and adjust to taste)
- A pinch of black pepper (to enhance turmeric absorption)
- Fresh mint leaves (optional for garnishing)

Instructions:

1. **Boil the Water**: In a small saucepan, bring 1 cup of water to a gentle boil.
2. **Add the Herbs**: Once boiling, add the ground cinnamon and turmeric (if using fresh turmeric, add it whole). Reduce the heat and let it simmer for about 5-7 minutes. This allows the beneficial compounds from the herbs to infuse into the water.

3. **Combine Ingredients**: After simmering, remove from heat, and strain the tea into a cup to remove any solid particles. If you used fresh turmeric, you may skip this step if you don't mind the texture.
4. **Enhance Flavor**: Add freshly squeezed lemon juice and honey (if desired) to taste. For an extra boost of health benefits, include a pinch of black pepper, as it enhances the absorption of curcumin (the active ingredient in turmeric).
5. **Garnish**: Optionally, garnish with fresh mint leaves for added flavor and a touch of freshness.
6. **Serve**: Enjoy your Cinnamon Turmeric Tea warm or let it cool and serve over ice for a refreshing drink.

Benefits of the Ingredients

- **Cinnamon**: Studies suggest that cinnamon may improve insulin sensitivity and reduce blood sugar levels in people with Type 2 diabetes. It also has anti-inflammatory properties that can help alleviate the risks associated with diabetes complications.
- **Turmeric**: Known for its powerful anti-inflammatory and antioxidant properties, turmeric may also help regulate blood sugar levels and improve insulin sensitivity.
- **Lemon Juice**: Rich in vitamin C and antioxidants, lemon juice can enhance overall health and may also assist in stabilizing blood sugar levels.

- **Honey**: While honey contains natural sugars, it has a lower glycemic index than refined sugar. Use it sparingly, and consider its effects on your overall carbohydrate intake.

Final Thoughts

While herbal remedies can offer additional support for managing diabetes, they should complement a balanced diet and a healthy lifestyle that includes regular physical activity and proper medical care.

Always consult your healthcare provider before incorporating new herbs or supplements into your routine, especially if you are taking medications that affect blood sugar levels.

Incorporating herbal teas and other natural remedies can be a flavorful and healthful way to enhance your diabetes management journey.

Cheers to good health and the healing power of nature!

19. Herbal Healing: A Natural Recipe for Managing High Blood Pressure

High blood pressure, or hypertension, is a condition that affects millions of people worldwide. Often dubbed a "silent killer," it can lead to serious health issues such as heart disease, stroke, and kidney problems if not managed properly. While conventional medicine offers various treatment options, many individuals are turning to herbal remedies as a complementary approach to promote overall well-being and manage their blood pressure.

Understanding High Blood Pressure

Before diving into our herbal recipe, it's essential to understand what high blood pressure is. Blood pressure is the force of blood against the walls of your arteries. It fluctuates throughout the day, but if it's consistently above the normal range (typically 120/80 mmHg), it may be classified as hypertension. Several factors can contribute to high blood pressure, including genetics, diet, stress, and a sedentary lifestyle.

The Power of Herbs

Many herbs have been recognized for their potential therapeutic effects on cardiovascular health. Some of the most promising herbs for managing high blood pressure include:

- **Garlic:** Known for its ability to relax blood vessels and improve circulation, garlic is believed to have a moderate effect on lowering blood pressure.
- **Hibiscus:** This vibrant flower has been shown in studies to help reduce systolic and diastolic blood pressure.
- **Cinnamon:** Commonly found in kitchens around the world, cinnamon may enhance circulation and help lower blood pressure levels.
- **Hawthorn Berry:** Traditional herbalists have utilized hawthorn for centuries to promote heart health and improve circulation.

Herbal Healing Recipe: Hibiscus and Garlic Tea

Ingredients:

- 1 tablespoon dried hibiscus flowers
- 2 cloves of fresh garlic, minced
- 4 cups of water
- 1 tablespoon honey (optional)
- A pinch of cinnamon (optional)
- Fresh lemon juice (optional)

Instructions:
1. **Prepare the Ingredients:** Gather all your ingredients. If you don't have dried hibiscus flowers, you can find them at a local herbal shop or online. Fresh garlic can be minced

or crushed for better flavor and health benefits.

2. **Boil Water:** In a medium-sized pot, bring 4 cups of water to a boil.
3. **Add Hibiscus Flowers and Garlic:** Once the water is boiling, add the dried hibiscus flowers and minced garlic. Reduce the heat and let it simmer for about 10 minutes. Hibiscus flowers will impart a beautiful red color to the tea while garlic adds a savory depth.
4. **Strain the Tea:** After 10 minutes, remove the pot from heat. Carefully strain the mixture using a fine-mesh strainer or cheesecloth, discarding the solid ingredients.
5. **Flavor it Up:** If desired, you can add honey for sweetness, a pinch of cinnamon for flavor, and a splash of fresh lemon juice for added vitamin C.
6. **Serve and Enjoy:** Pour the tea into cups and enjoy it warm, or let it cool and serve it over ice for a refreshing beverage.

Tips for Incorporating Herbal Remedies

- **Stay Consistent:** Include this herbal tea in your daily routine for the best results. Aim for 1-2 cups a day.
- **Balance Your Diet:** Combine this herbal treatment with a heart-healthy diet rich in fruits, vegetables, whole grains, and lean proteins.

- **Regular Exercise:** Engage in regular physical activity, as exercise can significantly lower blood pressure over time.
- **Monitor Your Health:** Keep track of your blood pressure readings and consult with your healthcare provider before making significant changes to your health regimen.

Final Thoughts

While herbal remedies can play a helpful role in managing high blood pressure, it's crucial to remember that they should not replace professional medical advice and treatment. Always consult a healthcare professional before trying new herbs, especially if you're already on medication for hypertension. By integrating herbal healing, a balanced diet, and a healthy lifestyle, you can take proactive steps toward your heart health.

Here's to a healthier you, naturally!

20. Herbal Healing for Autoimmune Disease: A Recipe for Wellness

Autoimmune diseases, conditions where the immune system mistakenly attacks the body's own healthy cells, can be challenging to manage. With symptoms ranging from fatigue and joint pain to cognitive issues, those affected often seek natural remedies to alleviate their discomfort and promote healing. Herbal medicine has been utilized for centuries in various cultures as a holistic approach to health and wellness. Let us explore an herbal healing recipe rich in anti-inflammatory properties that can support individuals with autoimmune diseases.

Understanding Autoimmune Diseases

Autoimmune diseases encompass a range of disorders, including rheumatoid arthritis, lupus, multiple sclerosis, and Hashimoto's thyroiditis, among others. While the precise causes of autoimmune diseases remain unknown, factors such as genetics, infections, and environmental triggers may contribute to their development.

Fortunately, natural healing methods can complement medical treatments and aid in managing symptoms.

The Power of Herbs

Herbs have been revered for their medicinal properties, with many offering anti-inflammatory, antioxidant, and immune-boosting effects. Some well-known herbs for supporting autoimmune health include:

- **Turmeric:** Contains curcumin, which has powerful anti-inflammatory properties.
- **Ginger:** Known for its ability to reduce inflammation and nausea.
- **Ashwagandha:** An adaptogen that helps the body respond to stress and modulates the immune system.
- **Nettle Leaf:** Rich in vitamins and minerals, it has anti-inflammatory and antihistamine properties.
- **Milk Thistle:** Supports liver health, which is crucial for detoxification and overall wellness.

Herbal Healing Recipe: Immune-Boosting Herbal Tea

This herbal tea combines the benefits of these powerful herbs to create a soothing and health-promoting drink. Consumed regularly, it may help reduce inflammation and enhance the immune system.

Ingredients:

- **1 teaspoon dried turmeric root (or 1-inch fresh turmeric)**

- **1 teaspoon dried ginger root (or 1-inch fresh ginger)**
- **1 teaspoon dried nettle leaf**
- **1 teaspoon dried ashwagandha root (optional)**
- **2 cups water**
- **Honey or lemon (optional for taste)**

Instructions:

1. **Prepare Your Ingredients:** If using fresh herbs, peel and thinly slice the turmeric and ginger. If using dried herbs, measure them out and set aside.
2. **Boil Water:** In a medium-sized pot, bring 2 cups of water to a boil.
3. **Add Herbs:** Once the water is boiling, add the dried turmeric, ginger, nettle leaf, and ashwagandha if you choose. Stir gently.
4. **Simmer:** Reduce the heat to low and let the mixture simmer for 10-15 minutes to allow the herbs to infuse.
5. **Strain:** After simmering, strain the tea into a cup using a fine mesh strainer or a tea infuser.
6. **Enhance Flavor (optional):** If desired, add honey or freshly squeezed lemon juice to taste.
7. **Enjoy:** Sip this herbal tea once or twice a day as part of your wellness routine.

Additional Tips for Managing Autoimmune Diseases

While herbal remedies can be beneficial, they should complement a holistic approach to health:

- **Mind Your Diet:** A diet rich in whole, anti-inflammatory foods, such as leafy greens, berries, fatty fish, and nuts, can foster overall health.
- **Stay Hydrated:** Drink plenty of water to support your body's natural detoxification processes.
- **Prioritize Rest and Recovery:** Stress can exacerbate autoimmune symptoms. Incorporate relaxation techniques such as yoga, meditation, or deep-breathing exercises into your daily routine.
- **Consult a Professional:** Always consult with a healthcare practitioner before starting any new herbal regimen, especially if you are on medication or have specific health concerns.

Final Thoughts

While autoimmune diseases can be complex and multifaceted, incorporating herbal remedies like the immune-boosting herbal tea outlined here can offer support. Remember, the journey to wellness is personal, and it's essential to find the right balance that works for your body. By accepting the power of nature and prioritizing holistic health, you can take proactive steps towards managing autoimmune disease and enhancing your quality of life.

Disclaimer: This recipe is not a substitute for professional medical advice. Always consult your healthcare provider before starting any new treatment, especially if you have an autoimmune disease or are taking medication.

21. Soothe Your Sleepless Nights: An Herbal Healing Recipe for Insomnia

Are you tired of tossing and turning in bed, counting sheep instead of getting the restful sleep you crave? Insomnia can be a frustrating and exhausting experience, impacting every aspect of your daily life. While modern medicine offers various solutions, many people are turning to nature for relief. Herbal remedies have been used for centuries to combat sleeplessness, providing a gentle and holistic approach to better sleep.

Understanding Insomnia

Before delving into our herbal remedy, it's essential to understand what insomnia is. Insomnia is characterized by difficulty falling asleep, staying asleep, or waking up too early. It can be caused by various factors, including stress, anxiety, poor sleep environment, and lifestyle choices. While it's essential to identify the underlying cause of your insomnia, incorporating herbal remedies can provide immediate relief and support your overall sleep health.

The Power of Herbs in Promoting Sleep

Herbs have been used for centuries in traditional medicine systems to promote relaxation and improve sleep quality. Some of the most commonly used sleep-inducing herbs include:

1. **Chamomile**: Known for its calming properties, chamomile works as a mild sedative, helping you relax before bedtime.
2. **Lavender**: Widely recognized for its soothing aroma, lavender can reduce anxiety and improve sleep quality when used in teas, essential oils, or pillow sprays.
3. **Valerian Root**: Often referred to as nature's tranquilizer, valerian root has been shown to reduce the time it takes to fall asleep and improve the quality of sleep.
4. **Passionflower**: This herb is known for its ability to reduce anxiety and promote relaxation, making it an excellent choice for those struggling with restless nights.
5. **Lemon Balm**: With its mild sedative properties, lemon balm can help reduce stress and promote calm.

Herbal Tea Recipe for Insomnia Relief

Now that we understand the benefits of these herbs, let's explore a simple herbal tea recipe that combines their powers for a soothing bedtime ritual.

Ingredients:

- 1 teaspoon dried chamomile flowers
- 1 teaspoon dried lavender buds
- 1 teaspoon dried valerian root
- 1 teaspoon dried passionflower

- 1 teaspoon dried lemon balm
- 2 cups of water
- Honey or lemon (optional, for flavor)

Instructions:

1. **Combine the Herbs**: In a bowl, mix the dried chamomile, lavender, valerian root, passionflower, and lemon balm. This blend not only promotes relaxation but also creates a fragrant aroma that enhances your pre-sleep routine.
2. **Boil Water**: Bring 2 cups of water to a boil in a small saucepan or kettle.
3. **Steep the Herbs**: Once the water has boiled, remove it from heat and add the herbal blend. Cover and let it steep for about 10-15 minutes. This allows the beneficial compounds to infuse into the water effectively.
4. **Strain the Tea**: After steeping, use a fine mesh strainer to remove the herbs from the liquid.
5. **Flavor to Taste**: If you prefer a sweeter taste, add honey or a squeeze of lemon. Both not only enhance the flavor but also provide additional calming properties.
6. **Enjoy Your Tea**: Sip your herbal tea about 30 minutes before bedtime to allow its relaxing effects to take hold as you wind down for the night.

Additional Tips for Better Sleep

Incorporating herbal tea into your nightly routine is just one step towards a better night's sleep.

Here are a few additional tips to enhance your sleep hygiene:

- **Create a Calm Sleep Environment**: Keep your bedroom dark, cool, and quiet to promote a restful atmosphere.
- **Limit Screen Time**: Reduce exposure to screens at least an hour before bed to help your mind transition into sleep mode.
- **Establish a Sleep Routine**: Go to bed and wake up at the same time every day to regulate your body's internal clock.
- **Practice Relaxation Techniques**: Consider adding meditation, deep breathing, or gentle yoga to your evening routine to further promote relaxation.

Herbal remedies offer a natural approach to combating insomnia, helping you to reconnect with restful sleep. With this soothing herbal tea recipe, you can take a substantial step toward improving your sleep quality. Remember, if insomnia persists or worsens, it's essential to consult a healthcare professional to explore the underlying causes and develop a comprehensive treatment plan. Embrace the power of nature and let its calming effects guide you to a night of peaceful sleep.

Sweet dreams!

22. Herbal Healing Recipe for Skin Burns: Nature's Touch for Relief

Skin burns can be a painful experience, whether they result from a kitchen mishap, too much time in the sun, or exposure to chemicals. While seeking professional medical attention is essential for severe burns, there are several herbal remedies that can provide significant relief for minor burns. These natural treatments have been used for centuries and can aid in soothing the skin, reducing inflammation, and promoting healing.

Understanding Burns and Their Impact

Burns are classified into three categories based on their severity:

- **First-Degree Burns**: Affect only the outer layer of skin (epidermis). Symptoms include redness, minor swelling, and pain.
- **Second-Degree Burns**: Involve both the epidermis and the second layer of skin (dermis). They may cause blisters and more intense pain.
- **Third-Degree Burns**: Extend through every layer of skin, potentially damaging underlying tissues. These burns require immediate medical attention.

For the purpose of this blog, we will focus on first and second-degree burns, which can often be treated effectively with herbal remedies.

Herbal Ingredients for Skin Burns

Certain herbs are known for their soothing and healing properties. Here's a list of some key ingredients you can use:

1. **Aloe Vera**: Renowned for its cooling and anti-inflammatory properties, aloe vera gel can speed up the healing process and provide relief from pain.
2. **Lavender Essential Oil**: Known for its calming scent, lavender oil is also an effective antiseptic that can promote faster healing and relieve pain.
3. **Tea Tree Oil**: With its natural antimicrobial properties, tea tree oil can help prevent infection and reduce inflammation.
4. **Calendula**: This potent herb has antimicrobial and anti-inflammatory properties, making it excellent for skin healing. It is often used in ointments and creams.
5. **Honey**: Raw honey has natural antiseptic qualities and can help in wound healing by keeping the burn moisturized and preventing infection.

Herbal Healing Recipe for Skin Burns

Ingredients:

- **2 tablespoons of fresh aloe vera gel**
- **1 teaspoon of calendula oil or infused calendula oil**
- **3-5 drops of lavender essential oil**
- **1 teaspoon of raw honey**

Instructions:

1. **Prepare Aloe Vera**: If using fresh aloe vera, cut a leaf from the plant and scoop out the gel into a clean bowl. If you're using store-bought aloe vera gel, ensure it is 100% pure without additives.
2. **Mix Ingredients**: In the bowl with aloe vera gel, add the calendula oil, lavender essential oil, and raw honey. Stir the mixture well until all ingredients are fully combined.
3. **Store in a Clean Jar**: Transfer the mixture to a clean glass jar. A small, dark glass jar is ideal to protect the oils from sunlight.
4. **Application**: Ensure the burn area is clean. Apply a thin layer of your herbal healing mixture directly to the burn and gently rub in. Reapply 2-3 times a day as needed.
5. **Patch Test**: Before applying the mixture extensively, conduct a patch test on a small area of skin to ensure there is no allergic reaction.

Additional Tips for Burn Care

- **Cool the Burn**: Immediately after a burn occurs, cool the affected area under running water for 10-20 minutes.

- **Avoid Ice**: Never apply ice directly to a burn, as it can cause further damage to the skin.
- **Cover the Burn**: Use a soft, sterile bandage to cover the burn to protect it from infection.
- **Stay Hydrated**: Drink plenty of water to help your body heal from any type of burn.

While herbal remedies can provide significant relief and promote healing for minor burns, always listen to your body. If a burn is severe or shows signs of infection (increased redness, swelling, pus), seek medical attention immediately. Using the power of nature, this herbal healing recipe can be a soothing and effective way to care for your skin. Embrace the wonders of herbal medicine, and keep your skin healthy and protected!

23. Herbal Healing Recipe for Pulled Muscles: Nature's Remedies at Your Fingertips

Getting a pulled muscle can be one of life's little surprises—usually at the most inconvenient times! Whether it's from an intense workout, a sudden movement, or just one of those quirks of life, the experience can be painful and frustrating. While conventional treatments like rest, ice, compression, and elevation (RICE) are essential, there are wonderful herbal remedies that can complement these methods, promoting healing and providing relief.

Understanding Pulled Muscles

Before diving into our herbal recipe, let's briefly understand what a pulled muscle is. This common injury occurs when a muscle or tendon is stretched or torn, sometimes leading to pain, swelling, bruising, and restricted movement. Recovery time can vary, but with the right care, you'll be back on your feet in no time.

Herbal Ingredients for Muscle Recovery

Several herbs are renowned for their anti-inflammatory, analgesic (pain-relieving), and muscle-relaxant properties. Here are some of the best options:

1. **Arnica (Arnica montana)**: Known for its ability to reduce bruising and swelling, arnica is a potent herb for easing muscle pain. Its anti-inflammatory properties make it a go-to for sprains and strains.
2. **Turmeric (Curcuma longa)**: This golden spice contains curcumin, which boasts powerful anti-inflammatory effects. It helps in reducing pain and swelling in muscles and joints.
3. **Ginger (Zingiber officinale)**: Ginger is another fantastic anti-inflammatory herb that can help ease muscle soreness.
4. **Comfrey (Symphytum officinale)**: Traditionally used in herbal medicine, comfrey is known for its ability to heal soft tissue injuries and promote cell regeneration.
5. **Eucalyptus (Eucalyptus globulus)**: This aromatic herb has anti-inflammatory properties and helps reduce pain when infused in oil.

DIY Herbal Healing Ointment for Pulled Muscles

Now that we have our herbal stars, let's create an easy yet effective DIY herbal ointment perfect for treating pulled muscles.

Ingredients

- 2 tablespoons of dried arnica flowers (or arnica oil)
- 1 tablespoon of dried turmeric powder
- 1 tablespoon of dried ginger powder (or fresh grated ginger if available)
- 2 tablespoons of dried comfrey leaves (optional, or comfrey oil)
- 1 cup of carrier oil (e.g., olive oil, coconut oil, or sweet almond oil)
- 15-20 drops of eucalyptus essential oil (for added relief)
- A glass jar for storage
- Cheesecloth or a fine strainer

Instructions

1. **Infuse the Oils**: In a double boiler, combine the dried arnica flowers, turmeric, ginger, and comfrey with the carrier oil. Gently heat over low heat for about 1-2 hours, stirring occasionally. This allows the properties of the herbs to infuse into the oil.
2. **Strain the Mixture**: After infusion, strain the mixture using cheesecloth or a fine strainer into a clean glass jar to remove the solid herbs. Be careful—the oil will be hot!
3. **Add Eucalyptus Essential Oil**: Once the infused oil has cooled slightly, add the eucalyptus essential oil and mix well.
4. **Cool and Store**: Allow the ointment to cool completely before sealing the jar. Store it in a cool, dark place. This infusion should last for several months if stored properly.

How to Use

To relieve muscle pain from a pulled muscle, apply a small amount of the herbal ointment to the affected area. Gently massage it in, allowing the healing properties to penetrate. Use this ointment 2-3 times daily or as needed for relief.

Caution

While natural remedies can be incredibly effective, it's essential to approach them with care. Always perform a patch test before applying herbal ointments to ensure you don't have an allergic reaction. Additionally, consult with a healthcare professional if the pain persists or worsens.

Pulled muscles can put a damper on your routine, but with the right care—both conventional and herbal—you can promote healing and enjoy relief. Our herbal healing recipe harnesses the power of nature's most effective remedies to ease pain and inflammation while encouraging recovery. So why not set aside a little time to create your own herbal ointment?

Your body will thank you, and you'll be back to your favorite activities in no time!

24. Herbal Healing: A Soothing Recipe for Nausea

Nausea is one of those unwelcome guests that can arrive unexpectedly, leaving you feeling uncomfortable and drained. Whether it's due to motion sickness, an unsettled stomach, or the aftermath of a delicious but perhaps overly rich meal, finding relief is essential. Luckily, nature provides us with a variety of herbs that have been used for centuries to ease nausea. Below, we'll explore a soothing herbal recipe that utilizes the healing properties of ginger, peppermint, and chamomile to help calm your stomach.

The Herbal Power Players

Ginger

Ginger is perhaps the most well-known herb for alleviating nausea. Its powerful anti-inflammatory properties and ability to stimulate digestion make it a staple in many traditional medicine practices. Ginger contains compounds called gingerols and shogaols, which can relax the digestive tract and reduce feelings of queasiness.

Peppermint

Peppermint is another fantastic herb for easing stomach discomfort. Its menthol content not only provides a cooling effect but also helps to relax the muscles in the gastrointestinal tract. This can lead to a noticeable decrease in nausea, making peppermint tea a go-to remedy for many.

Chamomile

Chamomile is often lauded for its calming effects on both the mind and body. It's anti-inflammatory, antispasmodic properties can help soothe the stomach and reduce cramping. Chamomile tea is an excellent choice for those moments when nausea is compounded by stress or anxiety.

The Herbal Healing Recipe

Soothing Ginger-Peppermint-Chamomile Tea

Ingredients:

- 1 tablespoon of freshly grated ginger
- 1 tablespoon of dried peppermint leaves
- 1 tablespoon of dried chamomile flowers
- 4 cups of water
- Honey (to taste, optional)
- Lemon (to taste, optional)

Instructions:

1. **Prepare Your Ingredients**: Start by grating fresh ginger and measuring out your dried herbs. The fresh ginger will provide a stronger flavor and more potent properties compared to dried ginger.

2. **Boil the Water**: In a medium-sized saucepan, bring 4 cups of water to a boil.
3. **Add the Ginger**: Once boiling, add the grated ginger to the water. Let it simmer for about 10 minutes. This will allow the ginger to infuse its beneficial compounds into the water.
4. **Add the Herbs**: After 10 minutes, reduce the heat to low and add the peppermint and chamomile. Allow the mixture to steep for an additional 5-7 minutes.
5. **Strain and Serve**: Remove the saucepan from the heat and use a fine mesh strainer to strain the tea into a teapot or individual cups.
6. **Add Sweetness and Zest**: If desired, add honey for sweetness and a squeeze of lemon for some brightness. Both honey and lemon have their own soothing properties and can enhance the overall flavor of the tea.
7. **Enjoy**: Sip your herbal tea slowly, allowing the warm liquid to work its magic on your stomach.

Tips for Best Results

- **Frequency**: You can enjoy this tea as often as needed, especially during bouts of nausea. However, if nausea persists, consult with a healthcare professional.
- **Herb Variations**: Feel free to adjust the proportions of the herbs according to your taste. Some may prefer more ginger for its sharpness, while others may enjoy a more minty flavor.

- **Other Additions**: Consider adding a pinch of cinnamon for added flavor and digestive benefits or even some fennel seeds, which can also alleviate bloating and gas.

Final Thoughts

Nausea can be an incredibly uncomfortable experience. While it's always essential to consult with a healthcare provider for persistent or severe nausea, many find relief through natural remedies. This ginger-peppermint-chamomile tea is not only easy to make but also a delicious way to soothe an upset stomach. Embrace the power of herbs and reclaim your comfort with this herbal healing recipe.

Cheers to good health and natural remedies!

25. Herbal Healing for Depression: A Natural Recipe for Wellness

In today's fast-paced world, mental health issues, especially depression, have become increasingly common. While traditional medicine plays a crucial role in managing symptoms, many people are turning to herbal remedies as complementary options to promote emotional well-being.

Understanding Depression and Herbal Remedies

Before we delve into the recipe, it's important to recognize that depression is a complex condition influenced by various factors, including genetics, environment, and lifestyle. While herbal remedies are not a substitute for professional medical treatment, they can provide supportive care and enhance emotional resilience.

Many herbs possess mood-enhancing properties due to their ability to interact with neurotransmitters, reduce inflammation, and promote relaxation. Some of the most well-researched herbs for managing depression include:

- **St. John's Wort**: Known for its antidepressant effects, it can help improve mood and relieve anxiety.

- **Ashwagandha**: An adaptogen that helps the body cope with stress and anxiety, promoting overall emotional balance.
- **Lemon Balm**: This gentle herb is known to elevate mood and reduce feelings of anxiety.
- **Chamomile**: Often consumed as a tea, chamomile can promote relaxation and improve sleep quality, assisting in overall emotional well-being.

Now, let's put these powerful herbs to use with a soothing herbal tea blend designed to uplift your mood and promote relaxation.

Herbal Healing Recipe: Uplifting Tea Blend

Ingredients

- 1 tablespoon of dried St. John's Wort
- 1 tablespoon of dried Ashwagandha root
- 1 tablespoon of dried Lemon Balm
- 1 tablespoon of dried Chamomile flowers
- 4 cups of boiling water
- Honey or lemon (optional, for taste)

Instructions

1. **Prepare the Herbs**: In a mixing bowl, combine the dried St. John's Wort, Ashwagandha, Lemon Balm, and Chamomile. Stir gently to blend the herbs thoroughly.
2. **Boil Water**: Bring 4 cups of water to a rolling boil.
3. **Steep**: Place the herbal mixture into a teapot or large heatproof bowl. Pour the

boiling water over the herbs and cover.
Allow the tea to steep for 10-15 minutes.
The longer it steeps, the stronger the flavor
and potential benefits.

4. **Strain**: After steeping, strain the mixture
   into your favorite teacup or mug, discarding
   the herb remnants.
5. **Add Flavor**: If desired, sweeten with honey
   or add a slice of lemon to enhance flavor
   and therapeutic properties.
6. **Enjoy**: Sip your uplifting tea slowly,
   allowing yourself to relax and enjoy the
   comforting warmth.

Usage Tips

- **Frequency**: Enjoy this tea one to two times
  daily as part of your self-care routine.
- **Mindfulness**: Engage in mindful sipping—
  focus on the flavors, aromas, and
  sensations as you drink. This practice can
  further enhance your relaxation and
  emotional state.
- **Consultation**: Always consult with a
  healthcare professional or herbalist before
  incorporating new herbs, especially if you
  are pregnant, nursing, or taking
  medications, as some herbs can interact
  with pharmaceuticals.

Herbal remedies can offer a gentle, natural
approach to supporting mental health and
emotional wellness. This uplifting tea blend
combines powerful herbs known for their mood-
enhancing properties, providing a soothing

experience for those facing the challenges of depression. While herbal healing is a wonderful addition to your wellness toolkit, remember that it's essential to seek professional help if you're struggling with severe depression or other mental health issues. A holistic approach—combining herbal remedies with therapy, physical activity, and a supportive network—can help you navigate your mental health journey.

Take a moment for yourself, brew a comforting cup of uplifting herbal tea, and embrace the gentle healing power of nature. Cheers to your health and well-being!

26. Herbal Healing for Staph Infections: Natural Remedies to Soothe and Heal

Staphylococcus aureus, commonly known as staph infection, can cause a range of illnesses from minor skin infections to more serious conditions. While conventional treatments are essential, many people seek herbal remedies to support their body's healing process. In this section, we'll explore an effective herbal healing recipe specifically designed to combat staph infections and promote recovery.

Understanding Staph Infections

Staph infections are caused by bacteria commonly found on the skin or in the nose of healthy individuals. They can enter the body through cuts, wounds, or areas of broken skin, leading to various symptoms like redness, swelling, warmth, and pain in the affected area. In some cases, staph infections require medical attention, especially when they turn into cellulitis or are associated with systemic symptoms.

It's important to consult with a healthcare provider when dealing with infections. However, integrating herbal remedies can be a beneficial adjunct to conventional treatment.

Herbal Healing Recipe: Staph Infection Salve

Ingredients:

1. **Calendula (Calendula officinalis)**
   o Known for its strong anti-inflammatory and antifungal properties, calendula promotes healing and soothes irritated skin.
2. **Tea Tree Oil (Melaleuca alternifolia)**
   o Renowned for its powerful antiseptic properties, tea tree oil can help kill bacteria and prevent infection.
3. **Garlic (Allium sativum)**
   o Garlic has natural antimicrobial properties that can combat a variety of infections, including staph.
4. **Coconut Oil (Cocos nucifera)**
   o This oil serves as a carrier and has its own antimicrobial properties, making it an excellent base for the salve.
5. **Beeswax (optional)**
   o To thicken the salve and create a more substantial consistency, beeswax can be added.

Instructions:

1. **Infuse the Calendula:**
   o Use about 1 cup of dried calendula flowers. Place them in a glass jar and cover with 1 cup of coconut oil. Seal the jar tightly and place it in a sunny spot for 1-2 weeks, shaking it daily. The heat from the sun will help infuse the properties of the calendula into the oil.

2. **Strain the Infused Oil:**
   o After 1-2 weeks, strain the oil through a fine mesh strainer or cheesecloth to remove the calendula flowers. You will be left with a vibrant, golden oil.
3. **Create the Salve:**
   o In a small saucepan, combine the infused coconut oil with 1-2 teaspoons of beeswax (if using). Heat it gently over low heat until the wax melts completely.
4. **Add Garlic and Tea Tree Oil:**
   o Crush 2-3 cloves of fresh garlic and add them to the mixture. Allow it to simmer on low heat for about 10 minutes to extract the garlic's properties.
   o Next, remove from heat and let it cool slightly before adding 15-20 drops of tea tree oil. Mix well.
5. **Store Properly:**
   o Pour the salve into small, sterilized glass jars and let it cool completely. Store in a cool, dark place.

Application:

- To use your homemade salve, apply it gently to the affected area 2-3 times daily. Make sure the skin is clean and dry before application.
- If you suspect a severe staph infection or it spreads, seek medical attention promptly.

Lifestyle Tips for Recovery

While your herbal salve helps to treat the infection externally, consider incorporating these practices:

- **Maintain Hygiene:** Keep the affected area clean and covered.
- **Healthy Diet:** A diet rich in whole foods, fruits, and vegetables supports your immune system.
- **Stay Hydrated:** Drink plenty of water to help your body fight off the infection.
- **Rest:** Give your body the time it needs to recover.

Herbal remedies can be powerful allies in the fight against staph infections, promoting healing and recovery in a more natural way. Our salve recipe combines potent herbs like calendula, garlic, and tea tree oil, harnessing their healing properties to support your skin's health. Remember that while these remedies can be effective, it's essential to work alongside healthcare professionals for proper diagnosis and treatment. Embrace the beauty of nature and its healing powers, and take proactive steps towards better health!

27. Embracing Herbal Healing: A Soothing Recipe for Menopause

As women journey through the various stages of life, menopause can be one of the most transformative—and sometimes challenging—periods. Characterized by a decrease in hormone production, this natural transition can bring a host of symptoms including hot flashes, night sweats, mood swings, fatigue, and insomnia. While many seek relief through hormone replacement therapies or over-the-counter medications, an increasing number of women are turning to nature's pharmacy: herbal remedies.

Understanding Herbal Remedies

Herbal remedies have been used for centuries across cultures for various ailments. Unlike traditional pharmaceuticals, these remedies typically rely on the synergistic effects of multiple plant compounds, providing holistic support for the body. When it comes to menopause, certain herbs are particularly beneficial due to their phytoestrogen properties, anti-inflammatory effects, and ability to help stabilize mood.

Key Herbs for Menopausal Relief

1. **Black Cohosh**: Renowned for its ability to relieve hot flashes and regulate cycles,

black cohosh is a staple in many herbal menopause formulations.

2. **Red Clover**: Rich in isoflavones, red clover can mimic estrogen in the body, helping to balance hormonal fluctuations.
3. **Chaste Tree (Vitex)**: This herb has traditionally been used for menstrual issues and is known to support hormonal balance and alleviate mood swings.
4. **Ginger**: Known for its anti-inflammatory properties, ginger can help soothe digestive issues that sometimes occur during menopause.
5. **Peppermint**: A refreshing herb, peppermint can aid in digestion and also provide a cooling effect to help with hot flashes.

Herbal Healing Recipe: Menopausal Relief Tea

This soothing herbal tea combines several of these powerful plants to create a warm, comforting drink that can be enjoyed daily to help alleviate menopausal symptoms.

Ingredients

- 1 tablespoon dried black cohosh root
- 1 tablespoon dried red clover blossoms
- 1 tablespoon dried chaste tree berries
- 1 teaspoon dried ginger root
- 1 teaspoon dried peppermint leaves
- 4 cups water
- Honey or lemon (optional, to taste)

Instructions

1. **Simmer the Ingredients**: In a medium-sized pot, bring 4 cups of water to a gentle boil. Add the dried black cohosh, red clover, chaste tree, ginger, and peppermint to the water.
2. **Steep**: Once the water reaches a boil, reduce the heat to low and let the mixture simmer for 10-15 minutes. This allows the flavors and beneficial compounds of the herbs to infuse into the water.
3. **Strain**: After the steeping time, remove the pot from heat. Use a fine sieve or cheesecloth to strain the tea into a teapot or directly into cups, discarding the solids.
4. **Serve and Enjoy**: Your herbal tea is ready! You can add honey or lemon for an extra flavor boost.
5. **Storage**: If you make a larger batch, the tea can be stored in the refrigerator for up to 3 days. Reheat as needed.

How to Incorporate This Recipe into Your Routine

- **Daily Ritual**: Develop a routine around your herbal tea. Consider sipping it each morning or evening as part of a self-care ritual.
- **Listen to Your Body**: Everyone responds differently to herbal remedies. Monitor how you feel and adjust the frequency of your tea as needed.
- **Consultation**: Always consult with a healthcare professional before starting any

new herbal regimen, especially if you are taking other medications or have pre-existing health conditions.

Navigating menopause doesn't have to be overwhelming. By embracing herbal remedies, you can find natural relief for some of the common symptoms. This soothing herbal tea recipe serves as a comforting daily reminder that you can take control of your health and well-being during this significant transition.

While this recipe may help ease discomfort, it's important to combine herbal remedies with a healthy lifestyle, including a balanced diet, regular exercise, and the support of friends and loved ones. Here's to embracing this new chapter with grace, resilience, and a dash of herbal magic!

28. Herbal Healing Recipe for Heart Palpitations

Heart palpitations can be an unsettling experience. Whether they feel like your heart is racing, fluttering, or skipping beats, they can be alarming. While it's crucial to consult with a healthcare professional to rule out any serious underlying conditions, many people find relief through natural methods and herbal remedies. Today, I am sharing an herbal healing recipe designed to support heart health and potentially alleviate palpitations.

Understanding Heart Palpitations

Heart palpitations can be triggered by various factors, including stress, anxiety, caffeine, alcohol, or even hormonal changes. In many cases, they can be benign and temporary, but they can also be a sign of more serious conditions. Listening to your body is essential, and if you experience frequent or severe palpitations, it's best to seek medical advice.

The Power of Herbs

Herbs have been used for centuries to support cardiovascular health. Many offer calming properties and can help regulate heartbeat and reduce anxiety. Below, I outline a simple herbal infusion recipe that combines several heart-friendly ingredients.

Herbal Infusion Recipe for Heart Health

Ingredients
1. **Hawthorn Berry (Crataegus monogyna)** – 1 tablespoon (dried)
     o Hawthorn is known for its ability to strengthen the heart and improve circulation. It can also help regulate heartbeat.
2. **Lemon Balm (Melissa officinalis)** – 1 tablespoon (dried)
     o This herb has calming effects and may help reduce stress and anxiety, contributing to fewer episodes of palpitations.
3. **Valerian Root (Valeriana officinalis)** – 1 teaspoon (dried)
     o Valerian is often used for its sedative properties, which can help soothe the nervous system and promote relaxation.
4. **Passionflower (Passiflora incarnata)** – 1 teaspoon (dried)
     o Passionflower helps calm anxiety and can aid in better sleep, both of which are important for heart health.
5. **Honey** (to taste)
     o Honey not only adds sweetness to your infusion but can also provide natural soothing benefits.
6. **Lemon juice (freshly squeezed)** – optional

- A splash of lemon juice adds flavor and can provide a boost of vitamin C.

Instructions

1. **Boil Water**: Start by boiling 4 cups of water in a medium saucepan.
2. **Add Herbs**: Once the water is boiling, remove it from the heat and add the dried hawthorn berries, lemon balm, valerian root, and passionflower.
3. **Steep**: Cover the pot and let the mixture steep for 20-30 minutes. This allows the herbs to infuse their beneficial properties into the water.
4. **Strain**: After steeping, strain out the herbs using a fine mesh strainer or cheesecloth.
5. **Add Honey and Lemon**: Stir in honey to taste and, if desired, a splash of freshly squeezed lemon juice.
6. **Cool and Serve**: Allow the infusion to cool before pouring it into a glass jar. You can store any leftover infusion in the refrigerator for up to a week.

How to Use

- **Dosage**: Drink 1 cup of this herbal infusion up to three times a day as needed. It's best to consume it in a calm environment where you can relax and enjoy the moment.
- **Listen to Your Body**: Pay attention to how you feel after drinking the herbal infusion. Adjust the frequency and quantity based on your individual needs and responses.

Additional Tips for Heart Health

1. **Practice Mindfulness**: Stress management practices like meditation, deep breathing, or yoga can be extremely beneficial in reducing heart palpitations.
2. **Limit Stimulants**: Consider reducing your intake of caffeine, nicotine, and alcohol, as all can contribute to increased heart rate.
3. **Stay Hydrated**: Proper hydration is crucial for overall health, including heart function.
4. **Maintain a Heart-Healthy Diet**: Incorporate plenty of fruits, vegetables, whole grains, and healthy fats into your diet.
5. **Consult a Professional**: If your heart palpitations persist, do not hesitate to seek medical advice. A healthcare provider can offer personalized recommendations.

While heart palpitations can be disturbing, integrating herbal remedies into your routine can offer natural support for your heart health. The blend of hawthorn, lemon balm, valerian root, and passionflower helps soothe both body and mind, promoting a sense of calm. Remember that everyone's body reacts differently to herbs, so it's essential to listen to your own needs.

Always consult with a healthcare professional before trying new herbal remedies, especially if you're already taking medications or have existing health conditions. Embrace this natural approach to healing and take a step toward nurturing your heart with the gentle wisdom of nature.

29. Revitalize Your Lymphatic System: An Herbal Healing Recipe

In today's fast-paced world, we often overlook the essential functions of our lymphatic system. This critical network of vessels and nodes plays a vital role in our immune function, detoxification, and general well-being. However, factors like diet, stress, and environmental toxins can hinder lymphatic flow, leading to a variety of health issues such as swelling, fatigue, and a weakened immune response. Fortunately, nature provides us with powerful tools for rejuvenating this system – herbal remedies.

Today, I'd like to share an herbal healing recipe specifically designed to support and stimulate lymphatic flow, promoting detoxification and overall vitality.

Understanding the Lymphatic System

Before diving into our herbal recipe, it's essential to understand why supporting the lymphatic system is critical. The lymphatic system is responsible for transporting lymph, a fluid rich in immune cells, throughout the body. This fluid collects waste, toxins, and unwanted material, filtering it through lymph nodes that help fight infection. When the lymph flow slows down, it can lead to a build-up of toxins, contributing to issues like lymphedema, chronic fatigue, and even skin problems.

Herbal Ingredients for Lymphatic Health

The following herbs are known for their lymphatic-cleansing properties and overall health benefits:

1. **Cleavers (Galium aparine)**: Often found in damp, shady areas, cleavers have traditionally been used to support lymphatic health. It's believed to enhance lymph flow and aid in detoxification.
2. **Red Clover (Trifolium pratense)**: Red clover is a powerful blood purifier with estrogenic effects. It helps to cleanse the blood and supports the lymphatic system.
3. **Dandelion (Taraxacum officinale)**: Often considered a weed, dandelion is packed with nutrients and known for its liver-supportive properties. A healthy liver contributes to better lymphatic function.
4. **Ginger (Zingiber officinale)**: This spicy root has powerful anti-inflammatory properties and can help stimulate digestion and circulation, facilitating lymph flow.
5. **Turmeric (Curcuma longa)**: Known for its active compound curcumin, turmeric is a natural anti-inflammatory and supports immune function.

Herbal Healing Recipe: Lymphatic Detox Tea

Here's a wonderful herbal tea infusion to encourage lymphatic health. This blend combines the supportive properties of the herbs mentioned above to create a delicious and healing experience.

Ingredients:

- 1 tablespoon dried Cleavers
- 1 tablespoon dried Red Clover flowers
- 1 tablespoon dried Dandelion root or leaf
- 1 teaspoon dried Ginger or 1-inch fresh ginger root, sliced
- 1 teaspoon ground Turmeric (or 1-inch fresh turmeric root, sliced)
- 4 cups water
- Honey or lemon (optional, for taste)

Instructions:

1. **Prepare the Herbs**: If you're using fresh ginger and turmeric, slice them thinly to help extract their flavors and benefits.
2. **Boil Water**: In a saucepan, bring 4 cups of water to a gentle boil.
3. **Infuse the Herbs**: Once boiling, add all the dried herbs (and fresh ginger and turmeric if using) to the water. Lower the heat and allow it to simmer for about 15-20 minutes. This process extracts the active compounds from the herbs.
4. **Strain**: After the tea has steeped, remove it from the heat and strain out the herbs using a fine-mesh sieve or a tea strainer.
5. **Serve**: Pour the herbal infusion into cups. Add honey or lemon to taste if desired. Enjoy your warm, nourishing tea!

Tips for Use:

- Drink this tea once or twice daily to support lymphatic health.

- Combine this herbal remedy with a healthy, balanced diet, regular exercise, and adequate hydration for optimal results.
- Consider incorporating dry brushing or gentle yoga to promote lymphatic drainage further.

The lymphatic system is a vital but often neglected part of our health. By nurturing it with herbal remedies, we can support our body's natural detoxification processes and maintain overall wellness. This herbal healing tea is a delicious and effective way to take care of your lymphatic system. As always, consult with a healthcare professional before starting any new health regimen, especially if you have existing health conditions or are taking medications.

Embrace the power of nature and give your lymphatic system the love it deserves!

30. Herbal Healing for Blocked Arteries: A Natural Approach to Cardiac Health

In our increasingly fast-paced world, heart health often takes a backseat to our busy lives. The problem of blocked arteries, a condition that can lead to serious cardiovascular diseases, has become a prominent concern. While medical interventions are crucial, nature has provided us with powerful herbs that can aid in promoting vascular health and potentially restoring arterial function. Here, we'll explore an herbal healing recipe aimed at supporting those with blocked arteries, alongside an overview of lifestyle adjustments and dietary tips for a heart-healthy life.

Understanding Blocked Arteries

Blocked arteries, or atherosclerosis, occur when plaque — a mixture of fat, cholesterol, and other substances — builds up in the arterial walls. This build-up narrows the arteries, restricting blood flow and increasing the risk of heart attacks, strokes, and other cardiovascular diseases. While it's essential to consult with your healthcare provider about medical treatments, incorporating herbal remedies into your routine may offer supportive benefits.

The Herbal Recipe for Heart Health

Ingredients:

1. **Turmeric** - 1 tablespoon (fresh or powdered)
2. **Garlic** - 3 cloves (minced)
3. **Ginger** - 1 tablespoon (grated)
4. **Cayenne Pepper** - 1/2 teaspoon
5. **Lemon Juice** - from 1 fresh lemon
6. **Honey** - 1 tablespoon (optional)
7. **Water** - 2 cups

Instructions:

1. **Prepare the Ingredients**: If you are using fresh turmeric and ginger, peel and grate them. Mince the garlic cloves.
2. **Combine Herbs and Water**: In a pot, bring 2 cups of water to a boil. Once boiling, add the turmeric, garlic, and ginger.
3. **Simmer**: Reduce heat and let it simmer for about 10-15 minutes. This will extract the beneficial compounds.
4. **Add Cayenne and Lemon**: After simmering, remove from heat and stir in cayenne pepper and lemon juice. Let it cool slightly.
5. **Sweeten (optional)**: If you prefer a sweeter drink, add honey to your mix, stirring until dissolved.
6. **Strain and Serve**: Strain the mixture into a glass. You can enjoy it warm or chilled.

How It Works

- **Turmeric**: Known for its active compound curcumin, turmeric has anti-inflammatory and antioxidant properties, which can help reduce arterial plaque and improve circulation.
- **Garlic**: Garlic is famous for its numerous heart health benefits, including lowering blood pressure and cholesterol levels, and preventing plaque formation.
- **Ginger**: This aromatic root supports digestion and has anti-inflammatory effects that can help protect the cardiovascular system.
- **Cayenne Pepper**: Contains capsaicin, which can help improve blood flow and circulation while reducing cholesterol levels.
- **Lemon Juice**: Rich in vitamin C and flavonoids, lemon juice promotes overall cardiovascular health and helps detoxify the blood.
- **Honey**: Not only does it add sweetness, but honey also contains antioxidants that further support arterial health.

Complementary Lifestyle Tips

While including this herbal remedy in your diet can be beneficial, it's essential to adopt a holistic approach to heart health:

- **Balanced Diet**: Incorporate whole grains, fruits, vegetables, lean proteins, and healthy fats such as olive oil and avocados

while avoiding trans fats and excessive sugar.
- **Regular Exercise**: Aim for at least 150 minutes of moderate aerobic activity each week. Walking, cycling, and swimming are all great options.
- **Stay Hydrated**: Drink plenty of water throughout the day to support overall bodily functions.
- **Manage Stress**: Practice stress-relief techniques such as meditation, yoga, or simple breathing exercises.
- **Regular Health Check-ups**: Keep track of your blood pressure and cholesterol levels with regular check-ups from your healthcare provider.

Blocked arteries can be a serious health concern, yet nature offers various herbs that can support heart health. Incorporating this herbal healing recipe into your daily routine, along with adopting a heart-healthy lifestyle, can provide protective benefits. Remember, always consult your healthcare provider before introducing new remedies or making significant lifestyle changes; they can provide personalized advice based on your unique health needs.

Welcoming a heart-healthy lifestyle today can pave the way for a more vibrant tomorrow!

31. Soothing Solutions: An Herbal Healing Recipe for Diaper Rash

If you're a parent or caregiver, you know that diaper rash can be a common yet uncomfortable experience for little ones. It can be caused by various factors, including prolonged exposure to moisture, friction, and even certain foods. While there are plenty of over-the-counter creams and ointments available, many parents are looking for natural remedies that are gentle and effective. Today, we'll explore an herbal healing recipe that harnesses the power of nature to soothe and heal your baby's delicate skin.

Understanding Diaper Rash

Diaper rash manifests as red, inflamed skin in the diaper area. It can make your baby feel uncomfortable and fussy, leading parents to seek immediate relief. Factors that contribute to diaper rash include:

1. **Wetness:** Diapers that are not changed frequently enough can lead to irritation.
2. **Friction:** Rubbing from the diaper can cause skin irritation.
3. **Dietary changes:** New foods can alter a baby's stool, leading to more acidic waste.
4. **Antibiotics:** These can disrupt the natural flora and lead to yeast infections, which can also cause diaper rash.

Regardless of the cause, the good news is there are natural remedies that can provide relief, one of which you'll find in our herbal healing recipe below.

Herbal Healing Recipe for Diaper Rash

Ingredients

- **1 cup of chamomile tea:** Chamomile is known for its anti-inflammatory and soothing properties. A warm chamomile tea can provide relief from redness and irritation.
- **1 tablespoon of calendula oil:** Calendula (or marigold) has powerful healing properties, making it a popular choice for wound care and irritation. Its antiseptic qualities can help prevent infection.
- **1 tablespoon of coconut oil:** Coconut oil is antifungal and hydrating, making it a great base for our healing mixture. It's known to trap moisture while providing a protective barrier on the skin.
- **1 tablespoon of shea butter:** This natural moisturizer is rich in vitamins A and E and helps to nourish and heal the skin.
- **Optional:** A few drops of lavender essential oil for its calming scent and additional healing properties (ensure you use pure, high-quality oil and avoid using it for babies under three months).

Instructions

1. **Brew the Chamomile Tea:**
   o Start by brewing a strong cup of chamomile tea. Let it steep for about 10-15 minutes, then allow it to cool to room temperature.
2. **Prepare the Herbal Mixture:**
   o In a small bowl, combine the calendula oil, coconut oil, and shea butter. Mix well until you have a smooth consistency.
   o If you choose to use lavender essential oil, add just a few drops to the mixture.
3. **Add the Chamomile Tea:**
   o Slowly incorporate the cooled chamomile tea into the oil mixture, stirring gently until fully combined. You should have a creamy, soothing balm.
4. **Transfer to a Container:**
   o Carefully transfer the herbal remedy into a clean, airtight container or a small jar for easy storage.

Application

1. After changing your baby's diaper, gently clean the area with water or a soft cloth. Pat dry; do not rub, as this can cause further irritation.
2. Apply a small amount of the herbal balm to the affected area, making sure to cover all irritated spots.

3. Use this remedy at each diaper change or whenever your baby shows signs of discomfort.

Additional Tips for Diaper Rash Prevention

- **Change diapers frequently:** Aim to change your baby's diaper as soon as it's wet or soiled to minimize moisture exposure.
- **Use breathable diapers:** Choose diapers made from natural materials.
- **Give diaper-free time:** Let your baby spend some time without a diaper to allow the skin to breathe.
- **Monitor dietary changes:** If you notice diaper rash after introducing new foods, consider whether those foods may be causing acidity in the stool.

Diaper rash can be distressing for both baby and parent, but natural remedies, like our herbal healing recipe, provide a gentle and effective way to alleviate discomfort. By using herbal ingredients known for their soothing and healing properties, you can promote your baby's comfort without exposing their sensitive skin to harsh chemicals. Remember, if the rash persists or worsens, consulting your pediatrician is essential for ensuring your little one gets the appropriate care. Trust the power of nature and provide your baby with the gentle relief they deserve!

32. Herbal Healing Recipe for Toothache: Nature's Approach to Relief

Toothaches can be excruciating. Whether caused by cavities, gum disease, or a cracked tooth, the discomfort can interfere with daily activities and sap your energy. While it's crucial to visit a dentist for long-term solutions, some herbal remedies can provide temporary relief for toothaches. We will explore an effective herbal healing recipe that harnesses the power of nature to ease your pain.

Why Herbal Remedies?

Nature has gifted us with a plethora of healing properties through various herbs and plants. Many cultures have relied on these remedies for centuries to alleviate ailments. For toothaches, certain herbs boast anti-inflammatory, analgesic, and antibacterial properties, helping soothe pain and combat infection.

An Herbal Healing Recipe: Clove and Peppermint Toothache Oil

Ingredients

- **5 whole cloves** (Syzygium aromaticum)
- **1 tablespoon of carrier oil** (such as olive oil, coconut oil, or jojoba oil)

- **2 drops of peppermint essential oil** (Mentha piperita), optional but adds a cooling effect
- **1 small glass jar with a lid** for storage

Instructions

1. **Prepare the Cloves:**
   - Lightly crush the whole cloves using a mortar and pestle or the bottom of a heavy glass. This will release the essential oils within the cloves, allowing for maximum potency.
2. **Combine Ingredients:**
   - In the small glass jar, combine the crushed cloves and your chosen carrier oil. The carrier oil acts as a base, allowing the clove oil to infuse and making it safe to apply to your gums.
3. **Infusing the Oil:**
   - Seal the jar and place it in a warm, dark spot for 24 hours. This will allow the cloves to release their beneficial properties into the oil. If you wish, you can let it steep for up to a week to enhance the potency.
4. **Add Peppermint Oil (Optional):**
   - If you choose to use peppermint essential oil, add two drops to the infused clove oil after the infusion period. Peppermint not only adds a delightful flavor but also helps provide a cooling sensation that can further ease discomfort.

5. **Strain and Store:**
   - After the infusion time, you can strain the oil (if desired) through a fine mesh or cheesecloth to remove the clove pieces, but it's not necessary as they can provide continued benefits. Store your herbal toothache oil in a cool, dark place.

How to Use

- **Application Method:**
  - To use your herbal healing oil, dip a clean cotton ball or a small piece of clean cloth into the oil. Gently apply it to the affected area of your gums/tooth. Be careful not to overapply, as concentrated clove oil can cause irritation. You can repeat this process every few hours as needed.
- **As a Mouthwash:**
  - Alternatively, you can dilute a few drops of the clove and peppermint oil mixture in warm water and use it as a mouthwash. Swish it around for a minute before spitting it out, which can help reduce pain and inflammation.

Additional Herbal Remedies for Toothaches

While the clove and peppermint remedy is effective, consider incorporating other herbal allies:

- **Saltwater Rinse:** Dissolve salt in warm water for a natural disinfectant rinse that can reduce inflammation and promote healing.
- **Garlic:** Crush a clove of garlic and apply it directly to the painful area for its natural antibacterial properties.
- **Turmeric Paste:** Mix turmeric powder with water to create a paste and apply it on the affected gums for its anti-inflammatory benefits.

Precautions

While herbal remedies can be effective, it's essential to remember that they are not a substitute for professional dental care. Persistent tooth pain could indicate a more serious underlying issue that needs evaluation by a healthcare provider. Always conduct a patch test before using new oils to check for allergic reactions, and consult your doctor before using essential oils, especially during pregnancy or if you have pre-existing health conditions.

Final Thought

Herbal remedies like the clove and peppermint toothache oil can offer temporary relief from the discomfort of toothaches while you await dental care. With their natural anti-inflammatory and antibacterial properties, herbs can be a soothing ally in your wellness journey.

Remember to listen to your body and seek professional help when needed.

Your smile—and overall health—deserves it!

33. Herbal Healing for Hearing Problems: A Simple Recipe to Support Ear Health

In an age where we are increasingly exposed to noise and stress, hearing problems are becoming more common. Whether it's age-related hearing loss, noise-induced damage, or ear infections, many individuals may benefit from natural remedies to support their auditory health. One such remedy is an herbal blend that leverages the power of nature to help manage and potentially alleviate hearing issues.

Understanding the Herbal Approach

Herbs have been used for centuries in traditional medicine to treat various ailments, including issues related to the ears. Specifically, certain herbs possess anti-inflammatory, antimicrobial, and antioxidant properties that can be beneficial for ear health. Before trying any new remedy, it's always wise to consult with a healthcare professional, especially if you have existing health conditions or are currently taking medications.

Key Herbs for Hearing Support

1. **Ginkgo Biloba**: Known for improving circulation, Ginkgo Biloba can enhance blood flow to the inner ear, which may support hearing function.

2. **Garlic**: Garlic is a powerful antimicrobial and anti-inflammatory herb. It can help prevent infections and inflammation in the ear.

3. **Olive Leaf**: This herb has strong antiviral and antibacterial properties, making it beneficial for combating infections that may affect hearing.

4. **Mullein**: Often used in herbal remedies for earaches, Mullein has anti-inflammatory and soothing properties, providing relief from discomfort associated with ear issues.

5. **Nettle**: Packed with essential vitamins and minerals, Nettle supports overall health and possesses anti-inflammatory properties that can aid in ear health.

Herbal Healing Recipe for Hearing Problems

Ingredients:

- 1 tablespoon dried Ginkgo Biloba leaves
- 1 tablespoon dried Mullein flowers
- 1 tablespoon dried Nettle leaves
- 2 cloves of fresh Garlic (crushed)
- 1 tablespoon Olive Leaf extract (or 1 tablespoon of dried Olive Leaves)
- 2 cups of water
- Honey (optional, for taste)

Instructions:

1. **Prepare the Herbs**: If using dried herbs, measure and combine the Ginkgo Biloba, Mullein, Nettle, and Olive Leaves in a bowl.

If using fresh Garlic, crush the cloves to release their beneficial properties.

2. **Boil the Mixture**: In a pot, bring 2 cups of water to a rolling boil. Once boiling, add the herb mixture along with the crushed Garlic.
3. **Steep**: Reduce the heat to low and allow the mixture to simmer for about 15-20 minutes. This allows the beneficial compounds from the herbs to infuse into the water.
4. **Strain**: After steeping, remove the pot from heat and strain the mixture into a heatproof container, discarding the herbs.
5. **Sweeten (Optional)**: If desired, add a teaspoon of honey to sweeten your herbal infusion. Honey also has additional health benefits!
6. **Consume**: Drink this herbal infusion 1-2 times a day. It can be enjoyed warm or at room temperature.

Additional Tips for Hearing Health

While this herbal remedy can be a supportive measure for hearing problems, there are other lifestyle choices you can consider:

- **Avoid Loud Noises**: Protect your ears by avoiding prolonged exposure to loud sounds, or wear protective ear gear when necessary.

- **Maintain Ear Hygiene**: Keep ears clean and dry to avoid infections that could impair hearing.
- **Stay Hydrated**: Drinking plenty of water helps maintain overall bodily functions, including ear health.
- **Nutritional Support**: Include foods rich in omega-3 fatty acids, antioxidants, and vitamins C and E in your diet to support circulatory and auditory health.

Natural remedies like the herbal infusion mentioned above can offer a supportive approach to managing hearing problems. However, it's essential to remember that these herbs should complement not replace traditional medical treatments.

If you experience persistent hearing issues, consult a qualified healthcare provider to explore comprehensive treatment options.

Embracing nature's bounty can bring us closer to holistic health, helping us to maintain our hearing and overall well-being.

Cheers to vibrant health and clear hearing!

34. Refresh Your Breath Naturally: An Herbal Healing Recipe for Bad Breath

Bad breath, medically known as halitosis, can be an embarrassing issue that affects our confidence and social interactions. While brushing, flossing, and regular dental visits are essential for oral health, nature offers some powerful herbs that can help combat bad breath organically.

Understanding the Causes of Bad Breath

Before we dive into the recipe, it's essential to understand what causes bad breath. Common culprits include:

- **Bacteria:** Oral bacteria break down food particles, producing sulfur compounds that lead to unpleasant odors.
- **Dry Mouth:** Saliva helps cleanse the mouth; reduced saliva flow can lead to bad breath.
- **Foods and Beverages:** Certain foods like garlic and onions, as well as beverages like coffee and alcohol, can contribute to a temporary odor.
- **Dental Issues:** Gum disease, cavities, and oral infections can also result in persistent bad breath.

Herbal Remedies for Fresh Breath

Herbs have been used for centuries to promote health and wellness, including oral health. Here are a few herbs known for their breath-freshening properties:

- **Mint:** Known for its strong aroma and flavor, mint can effectively mask bad odors and provide a refreshing taste.
- **Parsley:** Often used as a garnish, parsley is rich in chlorophyll, which helps neutralize odors in the mouth.
- **Fennel Seeds:** Fennel seeds have antimicrobial properties and a sweet flavor that can help freshen breath.
- **Clove:** This spice has antiseptic qualities and can be used to combat bacteria in the mouth.

Herbal Breath Freshening Recipe

Here's a soothing herbal tea recipe that can help freshen your breath while promoting oral health. This herbal infusion combines the beneficial properties of mint, parsley, fennel, and clove.

Ingredients:

- 1 tablespoon dried mint leaves (or a handful of fresh mint)
- 1 tablespoon dried parsley (or a handful of fresh parsley)
- 1 teaspoon fennel seeds
- 2 whole cloves
- 2 cups water
- Honey or lemon (optional, for taste)

Instructions:

1. **Prepare the Herbs:** If you are using fresh herbs, rinse them well in cool water. For dried herbs, measure out the quantities as listed.
2. **Boil Water:** In a saucepan, bring 2 cups of water to a rolling boil.
3. **Add Herbs:** Once the water is boiling, add the mint leaves, parsley, fennel seeds, and cloves.
4. **Simmer:** Reduce the heat and let the mixture simmer for about 10-15 minutes. This will allow the flavors and beneficial properties of the herbs to infuse into the water.
5. **Strain:** After simmering, strain the tea into a mug to remove the herbs and seeds.
6. **Add Optional Ingredients:** If desired, sweeten your tea with a small amount of honey or add a splash of lemon for extra flavor.
7. **Enjoy:** Sip your herbal breath freshening tea while it's warm. Aim to enjoy this tea 2-3 times a week for the best results.

Additional Tips for Combating Bad Breath

In addition to this herbal remedy, consider the following tips to keep your breath fresh:

1. **Stay Hydrated:** Drink plenty of water throughout the day to help keep your mouth moist and aid in flushing out bacteria.

2. **Maintain Oral Hygiene:** Continue to brush and floss daily, and don't forget to clean your tongue, as bacteria can accumulate there.
3. **Chew Sugar-Free Gum:** This can stimulate saliva production and help mitigate bad breath throughout the day.
4. **Avoid Odorous Foods:** Limit intake of strong-smelling foods, especially before social interactions.

Bad breath doesn't have to be a source of embarrassment. By incorporating this simple herbal tea into your routine, you can combat the issue naturally and effectively. Not only will you be freshening your breath, but you'll also be promoting your overall oral health with the goodness of nature. Remember, if bad breath persists despite these remedies, it's always a good idea to consult a dental professional to rule out underlying health issues. Sip your tea, breathe easy, and enjoy the refreshing confidence that comes from having clean, fresh breath!

35. Herbal Healing Recipe for Hair Loss: Nature's Remedy for Healthy Locks

Hair loss can be an emotionally challenging experience, leaving many people searching for effective solutions to restore their confidence and luscious locks. The good news is that nature offers many remedies that can help support hair health and potentially reduce hair fall.

Understanding Hair Loss

Before diving into our herbal remedy, it's important to understand some common causes of hair loss, which can range from hormonal changes, nutritional deficiencies, stress, and environmental factors. While consulting a healthcare professional is crucial for persistent hair loss, integrating natural herbs into your routine can be a valuable complementary approach.

Key Herbal Ingredients for Hair Growth

1. **Amla (Indian Gooseberry)**: Amla is a powerhouse of vitamin C and antioxidants. It helps strengthen hair follicles, promotes blood circulation to the scalp, and has anti-inflammatory properties that can soothe the scalp.

2. **Brahmi (Bacopa Monnieri)**: Known for its calming effects, Brahmi enhances blood circulation in the scalp, promotes hair growth, and reduces hair thinning.
3. **Fenugreek Seeds**: Rich in proteins and nicotinic acid, fenugreek seeds nourish the hair and strengthen roots. They also have antifungal properties that can help combat dandruff.
4. **Rosemary Oil**: This essential oil is reputed for its ability to improve circulation and stimulate hair follicles. It has also been shown to promote hair growth and prevent premature graying.
5. **Coconut Oil**: A natural moisturizer, coconut oil penetrates the hair shaft to reduce protein loss, keeping your hair healthy and hydrated.

Herbal Healing Recipe for Falling Hair

Ingredients

- **2 tablespoons dried Amla powder**
- **2 tablespoons dried Brahmi powder**
- **2 tablespoons fenugreek seeds**
- **1 cup coconut oil**
- **5-7 drops rosemary essential oil**

Instructions

1. **Prepare Fenugreek Seeds**: Soak the fenugreek seeds in water overnight. In the morning, drain the water and blend the seeds into a smooth paste.

2. **Combine Ingredients**: In a small, non-reactive bowl, mix the dried Amla powder, dried Brahmi powder, and the fenugreek paste.
3. **Infuse Coconut Oil**: In a small saucepan, heat the coconut oil over low heat. Be careful not to boil it; you simply want it warm enough to infuse the herbs. Add the mixture of powders and paste to the warm oil. Stir well and let it simmer for about 10-15 minutes.
4. **Add Essential Oil**: Remove the saucepan from heat and allow the oil to cool slightly. Once it cools, add the rosemary essential oil and mix well.
5. **Strain the Oil**: Use a fine mesh strainer or cheesecloth to strain the mixture, separating the oil from the solid herbs. Store the infused oil in a glass bottle or jar.

Application

1. **Pre-Wash Treatment**: Apply the herbal oil generously to your scalp, massaging it in to stimulate blood circulation.
2. **Leave It On**: Allow the oil to sit for at least 1 hour (or overnight for deeper nourishment) before washing it out with a gentle shampoo.
3. **Frequency**: Use this treatment 1-2 times a week for best results.

Additional Tips for Hair Health

In addition to using herbal remedies, consider implementing the following habits into your daily routine:

- **Healthy Diet**: Consume a balanced diet rich in vitamins (especially biotin and Vitamin E), minerals, and proteins that support hair health.
- **Stay Hydrated**: Drink plenty of water to keep your scalp and hair hydrated.
- **Reduce Stress**: Incorporate relaxation techniques such as yoga, meditation, or exercise to lower stress levels.
- **Gentle Hair Care**: Avoid excessive heat styling, tight hairstyles, and harsh chemical treatments that can damage the hair.

While individual results may vary, incorporating herbal remedies into your hair care routine can be a gentle, natural way to support your hair and scalp health. The combination of Amla, Brahmi, fenugreek, and rosemary in this recipe creates a nourishing elixir to combat hair fall. Always remember that consistency is key, and change takes time. Enjoy the journey to healthier hair with patience and care.

Unlock the secrets of nature and give your hair the nourishment it deserves!

36. Herbal Healing Recipe for Asthma: Nature's Breath of Fresh Air

Asthma is a chronic respiratory condition that affects millions of people worldwide. It can lead to difficulty breathing, wheezing, coughing, and tightness in the chest, which can be both distressing and challenging to manage. While conventional treatments exist, many individuals seek natural remedies to complement their medical care. Herbal healing offers a plethora of options, and in this section, we'll explore an herbal recipe designed to support respiratory health and alleviate asthma symptoms.

Understanding Asthma and Its Triggers

Before delving into our herbal recipe, it's essential to understand asthma better. Asthma is often triggered by allergens, environmental irritants, respiratory infections, or even physical exercise. Managing these triggers, along with a supportive diet and lifestyle, can significantly improve one's quality of life. While herbal remedies may not replace medical treatments, they can support respiratory health and overall well-being.

Herbal Ingredients for Asthma Relief

For this herbal healing recipe, we'll be using ingredients traditionally known for their anti-inflammatory and bronchodilator properties. Here are the key players:

1. **Thyme (Thymus vulgaris)**: A powerful herb recognized for its antimicrobial and anti-inflammatory benefits, thyme can help ease bronchial spasms.
2. **Ginger (Zingiber officinale)**: Known for its anti-inflammatory properties, ginger can help open airways and reduce inflammation in the lungs.
3. **Mullein (Verbascum thapsus)**: This herb acts as a soothing agent for the respiratory tract and can help expel mucus.
4. **Honey**: While not an herb, honey's soothing properties can help coat the throat and reduce irritation. It also has natural antibacterial properties.
5. **Peppermint (Mentha piperita)**: The menthol in peppermint can open the airways, making breathing easier.

Herbal Healing Recipe: Asthma Soothing Tea

This soothing tea combines all the aforementioned herbs and is designed to promote respiratory health and ease asthma symptoms.

Ingredients

- 1 teaspoon dried thyme
- 1 teaspoon dried mullein leaves
- 1 teaspoon grated fresh ginger (or ½ teaspoon dried ginger)
- 1 teaspoon dried peppermint leaves

- 1 tablespoon honey (raw, if possible)
- 2 cups of water
- Lemon slice (optional, for added flavor and vitamin C)

Instructions

1. **Boil Water**: In a small pot, bring 2 cups of water to a rolling boil.
2. **Add Herbs**: Once the water is boiling, remove it from heat and add the dried thyme, mullein leaves, and peppermint. If you're using fresh ginger, add it now as well.
3. **Steep**: Cover the pot and let the herbs steep for 10-15 minutes. This duration allows the beneficial compounds to infuse into the water.
4. **Strain**: After steeping, strain the tea into a cup using a fine mesh strainer to remove the solid herbs.
5. **Sweeten**: Add honey to taste, stirring until dissolved. You can also include a slice of lemon for added flavor and a boost of vitamin C.
6. **Enjoy**: Sip your herbal tea warm, ideally 1-2 times daily, or whenever you need relief from asthma symptoms.

Important Considerations

While this herbal tea can be a soothing addition to your wellness routine, it's vital to remember a few key points:

- **Consult with Healthcare Provider**: Always speak with your healthcare professional before integrating new herbal remedies, especially if you're already taking medications for asthma. Some herbs can interact with medications or may not be suitable for certain individuals.
- **Monitor Your Symptoms**: Keep track of your asthma symptoms and any changes you notice after incorporating this tea. It's crucial to recognize how your body responds.
- **Avoid Triggers**: Remember that this herbal remedy works best when combined with an overall healthy lifestyle that minimizes exposure to asthma triggers.

Asthma can be a challenging condition, but integrating herbal remedies into your holistic health regimen may provide comfort and support. The soothing tea recipe highlighted here not only tastes delightful but can also be a gentle ally in managing respiratory health. As always, staying informed and proactive about your health choices will empower you to navigate life with asthma effectively.

Breathe deeply, and embrace the healing power of nature!

37. Herbal Healing Recipe for Gallstones: Nature's Remedy for a Common Ailment

Gallstones are small, pebble-like substances that form in the gallbladder, a small organ responsible for storing bile produced by the liver. They can cause discomfort, pain, and other digestive issues when they obstruct the bile ducts. While medical intervention is often necessary in severe cases, many people seek natural remedies to alleviate their symptoms and promote gallbladder health.

Understanding Gallstones

Before diving into the herbal recipe, let's take a moment to understand gallstones. They typically fall into two main categories:

1. **Cholesterol Gallstones:** These are the most common type, formed primarily from hardened cholesterol.
2. **Pigment Gallstones:** These are smaller and darker, formed from bilirubin, a substance produced from the breakdown of red blood cells.

Those with gallstones may experience a range of symptoms including:

- Sudden pain in the upper right abdomen
- Nausea or vomiting

- Indigestion or bloating
- Jaundice (in severe cases)

Although lifestyle changes, such as diet and exercise, play a significant role in gallbladder health, herbal remedies can complement these changes, providing natural support.

An Herbal Healing Recipe for Gallstones

Incorporating specific herbs into your daily routine can support gallbladder function and potentially aid in the dissolution of gallstones. Here's a simple herbal tea recipe combining several ingredients known for their therapeutic properties:

Ingredients:

- **Dandelion Root (1 tablespoon):** Known for its ability to stimulate bile production and promote digestion.
- **Turmeric Powder (1 teaspoon):** Contains curcumin, which has anti-inflammatory properties and may help in bile flow.
- **Peppermint Leaves (1 tablespoon):** Soothes gastrointestinal discomfort and aids digestion.
- **Artichoke Leaf (1 tablespoon):** Supports liver and gallbladder health.
- **Lemon Juice (freshly squeezed from ½ lemon):** Aids in digestion and helps dissolve gallstones.
- **Honey (optional, to taste):** For sweetness and added digestive benefits.

Instructions:

1. **Prepare the Herbal Blend:**
   - Combine the dandelion root, turmeric powder, peppermint leaves, and artichoke leaf in a teapot or heat-safe container.
2. **Boil Water:**
   - Boil about 4 cups of water and pour it over the herbal mixture.
3. **Steep:**
   - Cover and let the blend steep for 10-15 minutes. This allows the herbs to release their beneficial compounds into the water.
4. **Strain:**
   - After steeping, strain the tea into cups or a teapot, discarding the solid herbs.
5. **Add Lemon and Honey:**
   - Stir in the freshly squeezed lemon juice and honey if desired for sweetness.
6. **Serve:**
   - Drink this herbal tea warm, ideally on an empty stomach or before meals.

Dosage and Frequency

Enjoy this herbal tea once or twice daily to support gallbladder health. However, it's always advisable to consult with a healthcare professional before starting any new herbal regimen, especially if you have existing health conditions or are taking medications.

Additional Tips for Gallstone Prevention

Alongside the herbal remedy, consider these lifestyle changes to further support gallbladder health:

- **Maintain a Healthy Weight:** Obesity can increase the risk of gallstones, so aim for a balanced diet rich in whole foods.
- **Incorporate Healthy Fats:** Instead of saturated fats, focus on healthy fats from sources like avocados, nuts, and olive oil.
- **Stay Hydrated:** Drinking ample water supports digestion and gallbladder function.
- **Regular Exercise:** Staying active can help maintain a healthy weight and reduce the risk of gallstone formation.

While herbal remedies like this tea can offer support for those dealing with gallstones, it's essential to approach the issue holistically. Always listen to your body, prioritize a healthy lifestyle, and seek medical advice when necessary. By incorporating herbal healing into your routine and making informed lifestyle choices, you can take proactive steps toward better gallbladder health and overall well-being.

38. Herbal Healing Recipe for Motion Sickness: Find Your Balance Naturally

Motion sickness can be a troublesome affliction, affecting anyone from casual travelers to avid adventurers. Whether you're experiencing nausea on a turbulent flight, a winding car ride, or a rocking boat, it can dampen the excitement of your journey. Luckily, nature has provided us with myriad herbal remedies that can ease these uncomfortable symptoms.

Understanding Motion Sickness

Motion sickness occurs when there's a disconnect between what your eyes see and what your inner ear senses. This dissonance leads to confusion in the brain, often resulting in symptoms like nausea, dizziness, sweating, and fatigue. While there are various over-the-counter treatments available, many people prefer looking toward natural remedies to alleviate their symptoms without the potential side effects associated with pharmaceuticals.

The Power of Herbs

Several herbs have been traditionally used to alleviate the symptoms of motion sickness, with ginger and peppermint being the most notable. Ginger is renowned for its anti-nausea properties, while peppermint is known for its calming effects on the digestive system. Together, they create a powerful combination that can soothe your stomach and help restore your sense of balance.

Herbal Healing Tea Recipe for Motion Sickness

Ingredients:

- 1 tablespoon dried ginger root (or 1 tablespoon of freshly grated ginger)
- 1 tablespoon dried peppermint leaves (or 1 tablespoon of fresh peppermint)
- 2 cups of water
- Honey (optional, for sweetness)
- A few drops of lemon juice (optional, for flavor)

Instructions:

1. **Boil the Water**: In a small pot, bring 2 cups of water to a boil.
2. **Add the Herbs**: Once the water is boiling, remove it from the heat and add the dried ginger and dried peppermint. If you are using fresh ingredients, add them at this stage.
3. **Steep**: Cover the pot and let the mixture steep for about 10-15 minutes. This allows the medicinal properties of the herbs to infuse into the water.
4. **Strain**: After steeping, strain the tea into a cup to remove the solid herbs.

5. **Customize Your Brew**: If you like, add honey for sweetness and a few drops of lemon juice for an extra zesty touch.
6. **Enjoy**: Sip the tea slowly, ideally about 30 minutes before your travel begins or at the first signs of motion sickness.

Tips for Use

- **Frequency**: You can drink this herbal tea as needed. It's great for preemptive use or as a remedy during travel.
- **Storage**: If you want to prepare a larger batch of this tea, you can store it in an airtight container in the fridge for up to 48 hours. Just remember to reheat it before consumption.
- **Travel Pack**: Consider preparing herbal tea bags ahead of time, so you can easily brew a calming cup while on the go.

Additional Natural Remedies

Besides the ginger and peppermint tea, several other methods can help with motion sickness:

- **Ginger Candies**: Chew on ginger candies or lozenges as they provide quick relief.
- **Acupressure**: Applying pressure to the P6 acupressure point, located a few inches above your inner wrist, can help alleviate nausea.
- **Stay Hydrated**: Drink water or herbal teas throughout your journey to keep your body hydrated.

Final Thoughts

Motion sickness can put a damper on your travels, but with this natural herbal remedy, you can find relief without relying on pharmaceuticals. Ginger and peppermint tea is not only soothing, but it's also easy to prepare and packed with health benefits. Next time you're hitting the road or taking to the skies, remember to bring along this calming herbal brew for a smoother journey.

Happy travels, and may your adventures be nausea-free!

39. Herbal Healing Recipe for Epilepsy: Nature's Touch for Balance

Introduction

Epilepsy, a neurological disorder characterized by seizures, affects millions of individuals worldwide. While medical treatments, such as anticonvulsants, have been vital in managing the condition, many people are also turning to complementary therapies, including herbal remedies, to support their health and well-being. Below we will take a look at an herbal healing recipe aimed at supporting individuals with epilepsy. Always consult with a healthcare professional before trying any new treatment, especially when dealing with a condition as complex as epilepsy.

Understanding Epilepsy and Herbal Remedies

Epilepsy results from abnormal electrical activity in the brain, resulting in recurring seizures. While the exact cause may vary—ranging from genetics to brain injury—individuals affected by epilepsy may seek ways to manage their symptoms and improve their quality of life.

Herbal remedies can sometimes work synergistically with prescribed medications to enhance well-being or reduce seizure frequency.

Certain herbs possess antiepileptic properties, while others help relieve anxiety or improve overall brain health.

Key Herbs for Managing Epilepsy

Before diving into our healing recipe, let's look at some of the key herbs often associated with epilepsy management:

1. **Passionflower (Passiflora incarnata)**:
   o Known for its calming effects, passionflower can help reduce anxiety, which may be beneficial for those with epilepsy.
2. **Brahmi (Bacopa monnieri)**:
   o An adaptogen, Brahmi is often used in Ayurvedic medicine to enhance cognitive function and may have neuroprotective properties.
3. **Valerian Root (Valeriana officinalis)**:
   o Known for promoting relaxation and sleep, valerian root can help manage stress, potentially reducing seizure triggers.
4. **Ashwagandha (Withania somnifera)**:
   o An adaptogenic herb that may help improve the body's resilience to stress, benefiting overall neurological health.

Herbal Healing Recipe for Seizure Support

Calming Herbal Infusion

Here's a simple herbal infusion combining several of the aforementioned ingredients that can be consumed regularly to promote relaxation and overall well-being.

Ingredients:

- 1 teaspoon dried passionflower
- 1 teaspoon dried Brahmi leaves
- 1 teaspoon dried valerian root
- 1 teaspoon dried ashwagandha root
- 2 cups of water
- Honey or lemon (optional, for taste)

Instructions:

1. **Boil Water**: Bring 2 cups of water to a rolling boil in a pot or kettle.
2. **Combine Herbs**: In a teapot or heatproof container, combine the dried passionflower, Brahmi leaves, valerian root, and ashwagandha root.
3. **Infuse**: Pour the boiling water over the herbs, cover the container, and let it steep for about 10-15 minutes. This allows the beneficial compounds in the herbs to infuse into the water.
4. **Strain**: After steeping, strain the infusion into a cup to remove the herb particles.
5. **Sweeten (Optional)**: If desired, add a teaspoon of honey or a splash of lemon juice for added flavor.
6. **Enjoy**: Sip on this calming herbal infusion once or twice daily, but be mindful of your

body's response and consult your healthcare provider.

Additional Considerations

While herbal remedies offer promising support, it's essential to remember the following:

- **Consult with a Professional**: Always consult a healthcare professional before introducing any new herbs, especially for individuals with epilepsy or those on anticonvulsant medications. Some herbs can interact with medications or have contraindications.
- **Monitor Progress**: Keep a journal of symptoms, triggers, and responses to the infusion to identify what works best for you.
- **Lifestyle Factors**: Incorporate stress-reducing practices such as meditation, yoga, and a balanced diet rich in whole foods to support overall health.

Herbs can be a valuable component of a holistic approach to managing epilepsy. Incorporating gentle, calming herbal infusions into your routine may offer additional support for relaxation and general well-being. Remember, each person's experience with epilepsy is unique, and what works for one person may not work for another. Always stay informed and prioritize your health in collaboration with healthcare professionals.

If you or a loved one is living with epilepsy, embracing natural remedies can be an empowering step toward managing this condition—finding the balance that works for you. Always listen to your body and prioritize safety on your healing journey!

40. Herbal Healing for Warts: A Natural Recipe to Promote Skin Health

Warts can be a bothersome skin condition, caused by the human papillomavirus (HPV). While they are typically harmless, they can be unsightly and even uncomfortable, leading many people to seek effective treatments. Instead of turning to over-the-counter medications or invasive procedures, you might consider a more natural approach.

Understanding Warts

Warts are non-cancerous growths on the skin that occur when HPV infects the top layer of the skin. They manifest as small, rough bumps and can appear anywhere on the body. Common types include common warts, plantar warts (found on the soles of the feet), flat warts, and genital warts. While most warts resolve on their own, they can take months or years to disappear, prompting individuals to seek quicker remedies.

Why Herbal Remedies?

Herbal remedies have been used for centuries in traditional medicine systems around the world. Many herbs possess antiviral, antiseptic, and healing properties that may help alleviate skin issues like warts. For those interested in natural solutions, several herbs show promising results in fighting viral infections, reducing inflammation, and promoting skin healing.

An Herbal Healing Recipe for Warts

Ingredients

1. **Apple Cider Vinegar (ACV)**: Known for its acetic acid content, ACV can help break down wart tissue and can also create an acidic environment that may be unfriendly to viruses.
2. **Garlic**: This potent herb has antiviral properties and contains allicin, which can aid in fighting infections.
3. **Tea Tree Oil**: Renowned for its antibacterial and antiviral properties, tea tree oil can help reduce the growth of warts and promote healing.
4. **Witch Hazel**: This natural astringent can help to dry out warts and reduce inflammation.

Recipe

Step 1: Garlic Paste
- **Ingredients**:
    o 2-3 cloves of fresh garlic
    o A small amount of olive oil or coconut oil (to create a paste)
- **Instructions**:
1. Peel and crush the garlic cloves into a fine paste.
    2. Mix with a small amount of oil to create a spreadable consistency.

3. Allow it to sit for 10-15 minutes to release its active compounds.

Step 2: Apple Cider Vinegar Soak

- **Ingredients**:
    - 1/2 cup apple cider vinegar
    - Warm water
- **Instructions**:

1. In a bowl, mix the apple cider vinegar with warm water.

2. Soak a clean cloth or cotton ball in the mixture and apply it directly to the wart for about 20 minutes.

3. Pat dry gently.

Step 3: Combining the Ingredients

- **Application**:
    1. Apply the garlic paste directly onto the wart after soaking in ACV.
    2. Secure it with a bandage to allow it to penetrate the skin.
    3. Leave it on for 3 to 4 hours, or overnight if possible.

Step 4: Using Tea Tree Oil and Witch Hazel

- **Final Application**:
    1. After removing the garlic paste, apply a few drops of tea tree oil directly onto the wart.
    2. Follow it up with witch hazel applied using a cotton ball. This will help soothe the area and reduce any irritation.

Frequency

- Repeat the soaking with ACV and application of garlic paste daily until the wart begins to diminish. The use of tea tree oil and witch hazel can also be done twice a day for added benefits.

Caution

While natural remedies are generally safe, it's essential to monitor your skin for any adverse reactions. If you experience increased irritation, swelling, or any unusual symptoms, discontinue use and consult a healthcare professional. Also, individuals with sensitive skin should perform a patch test before applying essential oils.

Natural remedies can offer promising alternatives for dealing with warts without the need for harsh chemicals or invasive procedures. The combination of apple cider vinegar, garlic, tea tree oil, and witch hazel can harness the healing properties of nature to help reduce your warts. Always keep in mind that consistency is key, and while some may see results relatively quickly, others may take longer to notice improvements. Always listen to your body and seek professional advice for persistent conditions or if you have any concerns. Embrace the power of herbal healing and let nature aid you in your journey toward clear, healthy skin!

41. Herbal Healing for Styes: A Natural Recipe to Soothe and Heal

Styes, often characterized by painful swelling and redness on the eyelid, can be both uncomfortable and frustrating. These small bumps, caused by clogged oil glands and bacterial infections, can disrupt everyday life, particularly when they affect our vision or appearance. While medical treatments are available, many people seek natural remedies to promote healing and alleviate discomfort.

Understanding Styes

Before diving into our herbal remedy, it's essential to understand what a stye is. A stye, or hordeolum, forms when a hair follicle at the base of an eyelash becomes infected. Symptoms typically include:

- A painful, swollen bump on the eyelid that may resemble a pimple
- Redness and irritation around the affected area
- Sensitivity to light
- Tearing or blurred vision in severe cases

While most styes heal on their own within a week, it's certainly helpful to have a natural remedy on hand to speed up the process and alleviate discomfort.

An Herbal Recipe for Stye Relief

The following herbal remedy uses ingredients that possess antibacterial, anti-inflammatory, and soothing properties. Before applying any herbal treatments, note that if your stye persists or worsens, you should consult a healthcare professional.

Ingredients

1. **Chamomile Tea Bags**: Known for their anti-inflammatory and soothing properties, chamomile can help reduce swelling and irritation.
2. **Warm Water**: To brew the tea and create a compress.
3. **Honey**: A natural antibacterial agent that can help fight infection and promote healing.
4. **A Clean Cloth or Cotton Ball**: For applying the compress.

Instructions
1. **Brew the Chamomile Tea**:
   - Take one chamomile tea bag and steep it in a cup of hot water for about 10–15 minutes. Allow it to cool until warm, but not too hot to avoid burning your skin.
2. **Prepare the Compress**:
   - Once the tea is at a comfortable temperature, take a clean cloth or cotton ball and soak it in the chamomile tea.

3. **Application**:
   - Gently place the warm, chamomile-soaked cloth over your closed eyelid where the stye is located. Make sure you're seated comfortably and in a relaxed position.
   - Leave the compress on for about 10–15 minutes. You can repeat this process several times a day, allowing your eyes to absorb the soothing properties of chamomile.
4. **Honey Treatment** (Optional):
   - For added healing, you can apply a small drop of honey directly onto the stye after the compress treatment. Honey can help fight bacteria and promote healing. Leave it on for 20-30 minutes, then gently rinse with warm water.

Additional Tips for Stye Prevention and Care

- **Keep it Clean**: Ensure that your eyelids are clean and free from oils and bacteria. Wash your face regularly with a gentle cleanser.
- **Avoid Eye Makeup**: Refrain from wearing eye makeup while a stye is present to minimize irritation and the risk of further infection.
- **Do Not Squeeze**: Resist the urge to squeeze or poke at the stye, as this can spread the infection.
- **Use a Warm Compress**: In addition to the herbal compress, a simple warm compress

with clean, hot water can help bring relief and encourage drainage.

Herbal remedies like chamomile and honey can provide gentle support in the healing process of styes, allowing you to find relief from discomfort and irritation naturally. While this recipe is effective for many, remember to listen to your body—if symptoms persist or worsen, seeking medical advice is always the best course of action. Enjoy the soothing power of nature, and may your eyes find comfort and clarity soon!

Disclaimer: This knowledge is for informational purposes only and is not intended as a substitute for professional medical advice or treatment. Always consult a healthcare provider for concerns regarding your health.

42. Herbal Healing Recipe for Hay Fever: Breathe Easy This Allergy Season

As the seasons change and spring blooms into full swing, many outdoorsy enthusiasts and nature lovers might find themselves battling one common adversary: hay fever. This allergic reaction to pollen can cause a range of uncomfortable symptoms, including sneezing, congestion, itchy eyes, and fatigue. While over-the-counter medications offer some relief, those looking for a natural approach can turn to the power of herbs. Below, we'll dive into an herbal healing recipe that has been traditionally used to help alleviate hay fever symptoms and promote overall well-being.

Understanding Hay Fever

Hay fever, or allergic rhinitis, occurs when the body's immune system overreacts to airborne allergens like pollen from trees, grasses, or weeds. With symptoms ranging from runny noses to headaches, it's easy to feel overwhelmed during allergy season. However, nature offers a toolkit of herbal remedies that could help ease these reactions without side effects commonly associated with pharmaceuticals.

Herbal Ingredients to the Rescue

Several herbs possess properties that can combat hay fever symptoms. Here are a few key ingredients you'll find in our herbal recipe:

1. **Nettle (Urtica dioica)**: Often used as a natural antihistamine, nettle can help reduce inflammation and relieve nasal congestion.
2. **Butterbur (Petasites hybridus)**: Butterbur contains compounds that block histamine release, making it particularly effective for allergy relief.
3. **Peppermint (Mentha piperita)**: Known for its soothing effects, peppermint can help clear airways and provides a refreshing aroma to ease your symptoms.
4. **Eucalyptus (Eucalyptus globulus)**: The steam from eucalyptus oil or infused leaves can help open nasal passages and ease respiratory discomfort.
5. **Honey**: Local raw honey is believed to help accustom your body to local pollens, potentially reducing allergic reactions.

Herbal Healing Tea Recipe for Hay Fever

Now let's get to the heart of the matter—a delicious herbal tea recipe that can help soothe your hay fever symptoms. This easy-to-make brew combines these powerful herbs to create an aromatic remedy that you can enjoy daily.

Ingredients

- 1 tablespoon dried nettle leaves

- 1 tablespoon dried butterbur (ensure it is PA-free for safety)
- 1 tablespoon dried peppermint leaves
- 1 tablespoon dried eucalyptus leaves or 2-3 drops of eucalyptus essential oil (if you prefer to brew without leaves)
- 1-2 teaspoons of local raw honey (to taste)
- 4 cups of water

Instructions

1. **Boil Water**: Bring 4 cups of water to a boil in a saucepan.
2. **Add Herbs**: Once boiling, remove the pan from heat and add the dried nettle, butterbur, peppermint, and eucalyptus leaves. If you are using eucalyptus essential oil, wait until the tea has cooled slightly (around 10 minutes), then add it in.
3. **Steep**: Cover the pot and let the herbs steep for 10-15 minutes. This allows the flavors and benefits to extract fully.
4. **Strain**: After steeping, strain the tea into cups, ensuring to discard the herbs.
5. **Add Honey**: While the tea is still warm, stir in the local raw honey until dissolved.
6. **Serve and Enjoy**: Sip your herbal tea slowly and relax. Feel free to enjoy 1-2 cups daily, especially in the morning and afternoon when pollen counts are typically higher.

Additional Tips for Managing Hay Fever

- **Stay Hydrated**: Drinking plenty of water can help thin mucus and reduce congestion.
- **Limit Outdoor Exposure**: On high pollen count days, consider staying indoors, particularly during peak hours (usually in the morning).
- **Keep Windows Closed**: Use air conditioning to filter out pollen and avoid letting it in through open windows.
- **Shower After Outdoors**: This helps remove any pollen that may have clinged to your hair, skin, or clothing.

Navigating hay fever can be challenging, but turning to nature can provide a refreshing and effective remedy. This herbal tea recipe is a gentle way to support your body during allergy season while embracing the healing properties of nature. Always consult a healthcare provider before beginning any new herbal regimen, particularly if you are pregnant, nursing, or taking medications.

Enjoy the beauty of springtime without letting allergies dictate how you feel—grab a cup of this herbal healing tea, relax, and breathe easy!

Happy healing!

43. Herbal Healing Recipe for Bronchitis: Natural Relief for Respiratory Health

Bronchitis, an inflammation of the bronchial tubes that carry air to and from the lungs, can often leave individuals struggling with persistent cough, mucus production, and general discomfort. While medical treatments are essential in managing more severe cases, herbal remedies can offer complementary support to bolster respiratory health and soothe symptoms.

Understanding Bronchitis

Bronchitis can be classified into two main types: acute and chronic. Acute bronchitis typically develops after a cold or respiratory infection, while chronic bronchitis is a long-term condition often caused by smoking or prolonged exposure to irritants. Common symptoms include:

- Coughing, which may produce mucus
- Fatigue
- Shortness of breath
- Chest discomfort
- Mild fever

Before trying any herbal remedies, it's important to consult with a healthcare professional, particularly if you have pre-existing health conditions or are taking other medications.

Herbal Ingredients for Bronchitis Relief

The following herbs are known for their potential benefits in alleviating bronchial discomfort:

1. **Thyme**: Renowned for its antimicrobial properties, thyme can help clear mucus and has antispasmodic qualities, which may ease coughing.
2. **Ginger**: A powerful anti-inflammatory, ginger can help reduce swelling in the respiratory tract and ease throat irritation.
3. **Honey**: While not an herb, honey is a natural demulcent, meaning it soothes mucous membranes and provides relief from coughing.
4. **Peppermint**: The menthol in peppermint helps to relax the muscles of the respiratory tract, promoting easier breathing and soothing swollen airways.
5. **Marshmallow Root**: Known for its mucilage content, marshmallow root provides a soothing effect on the throat and bronchial tubes.

Herbal Healing Recipe: Soothing Bronchitis Tea

Ingredients:

- 1 teaspoon dried thyme
- 1 teaspoon fresh grated ginger (or 1/2 teaspoon dried ginger)
- 1 teaspoon dried marshmallow root
- 1 cup of water

- 1-2 teaspoons honey (to taste)
- Optional: a few fresh peppermint leaves or a drop of peppermint oil

Instructions:
1. **Prepare the Herbs**: In a small saucepan, combine the dried thyme, ginger (fresh or dried), and marshmallow root.
2. **Boil the Water**: Add 1 cup of water to the saucepan and bring it to a boil.
3. **Simmer**: Once boiling, reduce the heat and let the mixture simmer for about 10-15 minutes. This allows the herbs to release their beneficial properties fully.
4. **Strain**: After simmering, strain the tea through a fine mesh sieve into a cup to remove the solid herbs.
5. **Add Honey and Peppermint**: Add honey to taste for sweetness and, if desired, a few fresh peppermint leaves or a drop of peppermint oil for added flavor and soothing benefits.
6. **Serve and Sip**: Drink the tea while it's warm for the best soothing effect. Aim for 1-2 cups per day, especially during times of increased bronchial discomfort.

Additional Tips for Managing Bronchitis Naturally

- **Stay Hydrated**: Drink plenty of fluids to help thin mucus and promote easier breathing.
- **Steam Inhalation**: Inhaling steam from a hot shower or bowl of hot water can provide

further relief by moistening irritated
airways.
- **Rest**: Give your body time to heal; adequate
rest is vital during any respiratory illness.
- **Humidifier**: Use a humidifier in your home
to keep the air moist, helping to ease cough
and congestion.

Final Thoughts

Herbal remedies can be a gentle and effective way
to support your body during bouts of bronchitis.
However, it's crucial to remember that herbal
remedies should complement, not replace,
medical treatment. Monitor your symptoms, and
if they worsen or do not improve, consult a
healthcare professional.

Always prioritize your health, and consider
incorporating this soothing herbal tea recipe into
your routine when facing respiratory distress.
May your bronchial health improve and your path
to recovery be swift!

44. Herbal Healing for Low Blood Pressure: A Soothing Recipe

Low blood pressure, also known as hypotension, can leave you feeling dizzy, weak, and fatigued. While it's often less talked about than hypertension, it's a condition that can significantly affect your quality of life. Fortunately, nature provides us with a wealth of healing herbs that can help manage low blood pressure symptoms effectively and safely.

Understanding Low Blood Pressure

Before we dive into our herbal recipe, let's briefly discuss what low blood pressure is. Hypotension is generally defined as blood pressure below 90/60 mmHg. Symptoms might include:

- Dizziness or lightheadedness
- Fainting
- Nausea
- Fatigue
- Blurred vision

Lifestyle factors, medications, pregnancy, and underlying health issues can contribute to low blood pressure. Always consult a healthcare professional if you are concerned about your blood pressure levels.

Herbal Healing Recipe: Adaptogenic Tonic

Ingredients:

- **2 cups of water**
- **1 tablespoon of dried nettle leaf**: Nettle is rich in iron and vitamins and can help strengthen the bloodstream.
- **1 tablespoon of ashwagandha**: This adaptogenic herb can support adrenal health and help your body adapt to stress.
- **1 tablespoon of licorice root**: Licorice helps increase blood pressure and add a natural sweetness to the tonic.
- **1 tablespoon of rosemary**: This herb not only adds flavor but can also stimulate circulation and improve overall vascular health.
- **Honey** (to taste): A natural sweetener that provides additional nutrients.

Instructions:

1. **Boil the Water**: In a medium saucepan, bring 2 cups of water to a boil.
2. **Add the Herbs**: Once boiling, reduce heat and add dried nettle leaf, ashwagandha, licorice root, and rosemary. Stir well to combine.
3. **Simmer**: Cover the pot and let the mixture simmer on low heat for about 15-20 minutes. This allows the beneficial compounds in the herbs to infuse into the water.
4. **Strain the Mixture**: After simmering, strain the tonic through a fine-mesh sieve

or cheesecloth into a clean container. Discard the herbal material.

5. **Sweeten**: While the tonic is still warm, add honey to taste. Stir until it's fully dissolved.
6. **Cool and Store**: Let the tonic cool completely. You can store it in the refrigerator for up to one week. Consume ½ cup daily, either warm or cold.

Additional Tips:

- **Stay Hydrated**: Drink plenty of fluids, especially water, to help maintain blood volume and prevent dehydration, which can exacerbate low blood pressure.
- **Eat Small Meals**: Large meals can contribute to a drop in blood pressure, so consider smaller, more frequent meals throughout the day.
- **Incorporate Physical Activity**: Light exercises like walking or yoga can improve circulation and overall cardiovascular health.

Caution:

While herbal remedies can be effective, it's crucial to consult with a healthcare provider before starting any new supplement or treatment, especially if you are pregnant, nursing, or taking medications.

Herbal healing offers a natural, holistic approach to managing low blood pressure. This adaptogenic tonic combines synergistic herbs known for their beneficial properties and can help uplift your energy levels and stabilize your blood pressure. Your health is a balance of body, mind, and spirit; embrace these natural remedies as part of a lifestyle that nurtures all aspects of your well-being.

Stay healthy, stay inspired, and let nature's gifts support you on your wellness journey!

45. Natural Remedies: An Herbal Healing Recipe for Intestinal Parasites

Introduction

In today's world, our bodies are constantly exposed to various toxins and harmful microorganisms, including intestinal parasites. These unwelcome guests can lead to a range of health issues, from digestive problems to fatigue. Thankfully, nature provides us with an array of herbal remedies that can help cleanse our bodies of these parasites and restore our well-being.

Understanding Intestinal Parasites

Intestinal parasites, such as Giardia, roundworms, and tapeworms, can enter our bodies through contaminated food, water, or even through contact with infected individuals. Symptoms may include abdominal pain, bloating, diarrhea, fatigue, and unexplained weight loss. While conventional medicine is effective in treating these infections, many people are turning to natural remedies as a complementary approach to healing.

Herbal Ingredients for Parasite Cleansing

Before we dive into our herbal healing recipe, let's look at some of the most effective herbs for combating intestinal parasites:

1. **Wormwood (Artemisia absinthium)**: Known for its bitter properties, wormwood is traditionally used to expel worms and parasites from the intestines.
2. **Black Walnut (Juglans nigra)**: The hulls of this nut have antifungal and antiparasitic properties, making it a potent tool in the fight against parasites.
3. **Clove (Syzygium aromaticum)**: Cloves contain compounds that may help neutralize adult parasites and their eggs, preventing further infection.
4. **Garlic (Allium sativum)**: This common kitchen herb is renowned for its antimicrobial properties and can help eliminate parasites while enhancing immune function.
5. **Ginger (Zingiber officinale)**: Ginger has anti-inflammatory properties and aids in digestion, making it an excellent addition to any parasite cleanse.

Herbal Healing Recipe for Intestinal Parasites

Ingredients:

- 1 teaspoon dried wormwood
- 1 teaspoon black walnut hull powder
- 1 teaspoon ground cloves
- 2 cloves of fresh garlic, minced
- 1 tablespoon fresh ginger, grated

- 2 cups water
- Raw honey (optional, to taste)
- Fresh lemon juice (optional, for flavor)

Instructions:

1. **Prepare the Herbal Tea:**
   - Start by boiling the water in a pot.
   - Once the water reaches a rolling boil, add the wormwood, black walnut hull powder, and ground cloves.
   - Reduce the heat and let the mixture simmer for about 10-15 minutes. This allows the herbs to release their beneficial compounds into the water.
2. **Add Garlic and Ginger:**
   - After simmering, remove the pot from heat and add the minced garlic and grated ginger to the herbal infusion. Cover and let it steep for an additional 10 minutes. This step boosts the antimicrobial properties of the remedy.
3. **Strain and Serve:**
   - Strain the herbal mixture into a cup, discarding the solids. If desired, sweeten your tea with raw honey and add a splash of fresh lemon juice for flavor and extra vitamin C.
4. **Dosage:**
   - Drink this herbal tea once a day for one to two weeks. Remember to consult with a healthcare professional before beginning any herbal regimen, especially if you are

pregnant, nursing, or taking
medications.

Herbal remedies have been used for centuries to
support the body in its natural healing processes.
The combination of wormwood, black walnut,
cloves, garlic, and ginger creates a powerful
potion against intestinal parasites while
supporting digestive health.

However, it's essential to remember that while
herbal remedies can be effective, they should
complement a healthy lifestyle. Ensure a
balanced diet, stay hydrated, and practice good
hygiene to help prevent parasites in the first
place.

46. Herbal Healing Recipe for Dandruff: Banish Flakes Naturally

Dandruff is a common scalp condition that can be both annoying and embarrassing. It is characterized by flaky skin on the scalp, often accompanied by itchiness and dryness. While there are many commercial products available to combat dandruff, herbal remedies offer a natural, gentle alternative.

Understanding Dandruff

Before we dive into the remedy, it's helpful to understand what causes dandruff. There are several factors that contribute to this condition, including:

- **Dry Skin:** Cold, dry weather can cause your scalp to lose moisture.
- **Seborrheic Dermatitis:** This more severe form of dandruff involves inflamed and oily skin, which leads to yellow or white flakes.
- **Fungal Infections:** A yeast-like fungus called Malassezia can affect the scalp, causing irritation and flaking.
- **Sensitivity to Hair Products:** Allergic reactions or sensitivity to hair care products can also result in dandruff.

Herbal Healing Recipe for Dandruff: DIY Herbal Rinse

This all-natural herbal rinse harnesses the power of essential oils and herbal extracts known for their anti-inflammatory and antifungal properties. Here's what you will need:

Ingredients:

- **2 cups of water**
- **2 tablespoons dried rosemary leaves**
- **2 tablespoons dried nettle leaves**
- **2 tablespoons dried chamomile flowers**
- **2 tablespoons apple cider vinegar**
- **10 drops of tea tree essential oil**
- **10 drops of lavender essential oil**

Instructions:

1. **Prepare the Herbal Infusion:**
   - In a pot, bring 2 cups of water to a boil.
   - Once boiling, remove from heat and add the dried rosemary, nettle, and chamomile.
   - Cover and let it steep for about 20-30 minutes. The herbs will infuse their beneficial properties into the water.
2. **Strain the Mixture:**
   - After steeping, strain the herbal infusion into a clean bowl or container to remove the plant material.
3. **Add the Vinegar and Essential Oils:**
   - Allow the infusion to cool slightly before adding the apple cider vinegar, tea tree oil, and lavender oil. Stir gently to combine.

4. **Storage:**
    o   Pour the mixture into a clean glass
        bottle. You can store this herbal rinse
        in the refrigerator for up to one week.

How to Use the Herbal Rinse:

1. **Shampoo First:** Start by washing your hair
   with a gentle shampoo to remove dirt and
   excess oils.
2. **Apply the Rinse:** After rinsing out the
   shampoo, pour the herbal rinse over your
   scalp, ensuring that you cover the entire
   area. You can massage it lightly into your
   scalp for better absorption.
3. **Let It Sit:** Allow the herbal rinse to sit on
   your scalp for about 5-10 minutes. During
   this time, you can relax and enjoy the
   soothing fragrance of the herbs.
4. **Rinse Out (Optional):** If you find the
   vinegar smell too strong, you can rinse it
   out with water. However, for best results,
   leaving it in can continue to nourish and
   balance your scalp.
5. **Frequency:** Use this rinse 1-2 times a week
   or whenever you wash your hair for optimal
   results.

Benefits of the Ingredients:

- **Rosemary:** Known for its ability to
  stimulate circulation, rosemary can
  promote healthy hair growth while its
  antifungal properties help fight dandruff.

- **Nettle:** Rich in vitamins and minerals, nettle is excellent for scalp health and can help to reduce inflammation.
- **Chamomile:** This calming herb is anti-inflammatory, soothing itchy and irritated skin.
- **Apple Cider Vinegar:** ACV helps to restore the pH balance of the scalp, while its antifungal properties can combat the growth of Malassezia.
- **Tea Tree Oil:** Renowned for its powerful antifungal capabilities, tea tree oil can address the underlying causes of dandruff.
- **Lavender Oil:** Beyond its pleasant aroma, lavender oil has anti-inflammatory properties that can help sooth irritated skin.

Final Thoughts

If you are struggling with dandruff, this herbal rinse may be the natural solution you've been looking for. The ingredients are not only beneficial for combating flakes, but they also promote overall scalp health. As with any new treatment, remember to patch-test first to ensure you don't have sensitivity to any of the ingredients. Embrace the healing powers of nature and enjoy a flake-free, healthy scalp!

47. Herbal Healing Recipe for Varicose Ulcers

Varicose ulcers are a frustrating and painful condition that can arise from chronic venous insufficiency, where the veins struggle to return blood to the heart. This can lead to swelling, discoloration, and eventually, the formation of ulcers. While conventional treatments are available, many individuals are turning to herbal remedies for a more holistic approach to healing. Today, we will explore an herbal healing recipe designed to support the healing of varicose ulcers and promote overall skin health.

Understanding Varicose Ulcers

Before diving into our herbal recipe, it is essential to understand the condition. Varicose ulcers usually occur on the lower legs and can result in open sores that are slow to heal. They often present with symptoms such as pain, itching, and a feeling of heaviness in the affected area. While it's crucial to consult with a healthcare professional regarding proper diagnosis and treatment, herbal remedies can serve as a complementary approach.

Herbal Ingredients for Healing

When formulating an herbal remedy for varicose ulcers, certain herbs are particularly beneficial due to their anti-inflammatory, antimicrobial, and wound-healing properties. Here are a few key ingredients to consider:

1. **Calendula (Calendula officinalis)**: Known for its superb healing properties, calendula promotes tissue regeneration and has anti-inflammatory characteristics. It helps soothe irritated skin and fights infection.
2. **Comfrey (Symphytum officinale)**: This herb is traditionally used to support wound healing. Comfrey contains allantoin, a compound that encourages cell regeneration and reduces inflammation.
3. **Witch Hazel (Hamamelis virginiana)**: Often used for its astringent properties, witch hazel can improve blood circulation and reduce swelling, making it a great choice for varicose veins and ulcers.
4. **Chamomile (Matricaria chamomilla)**: This calming herb is effective in reducing inflammation and promoting relaxation. Its antibacterial properties also make it a valuable addition for wound care.
5. **Hypericum (St. John's Wort)**: Known for its ability to soothe nerve pain and promote healing, Hypericum is effective against inflammation and infection.

Now, let's look at a simple herbal remedy that combines these powerful ingredients.

Herbal Salve for Varicose Ulcers

Ingredients

- 2 tablespoons dried calendula flowers
- 2 tablespoons dried comfrey root
- 2 tablespoons dried chamomile flowers
- 1 tablespoon dried Hypericum (St. John's Wort)
- 1 cup olive oil (or coconut oil as an alternative)
- 1 ounce beeswax (optional, for thicker salve)
- A few drops of lavender essential oil (optional, for fragrance and additional healing properties)

Instructions

1. **Infuse the Herbal Oil**:
   - In a double boiler or a small saucepan, combine the dried herbs and olive oil. Gently heat the mixture over low heat for 2-3 hours, allowing the herbs to infuse their properties into the oil. Ensure that the oil does not reach a boiling point.
2. **Strain the Mixture**:
   - After the infusion period, remove the oil from heat and let it cool slightly. Strain the oil using a fine mesh strainer or cheesecloth to remove the herbal solids.
3. **Create the Salve**:
   - If you prefer a thicker consistency, return the strained oil to the double

boiler, add the beeswax, and stir
until melted and fully integrated.
  o Remove from heat and let it cool for a
    few minutes before adding lavender
    essential oil.
4. **Store the Salve**:
  o Pour the mixture into small, clean
    jars or tins and allow it to cool
    completely. Seal and store in a cool,
    dark place.

Application

To use the herbal salve, clean the affected area
gently and apply a thin layer of the salve directly
onto the ulcer. Cover it with a sterile bandage if
necessary. For best results, apply the salve twice
daily until healing occurs.

Safety Precautions

- Always conduct a patch test on a small area
  of skin before using any new herbal
  remedy to ensure there are no adverse
  reactions.
- Consult with a healthcare professional to
  discuss any potential interactions,
  particularly if you are on medication or
  have underlying health conditions.
- If symptoms worsen or do not improve, seek
  medical advice.

Herbal remedies can provide a natural
complement to traditional treatments for varicose
ulcers. This herbal salve, infused with powerful

healing ingredients, not only helps to soothe the skin but also supports the natural healing process. Remember that while herbal remedies can be beneficial, they should not replace medical advice or treatment. Embrace a holistic approach to healing, and may you find comfort and relief on your journey to wellness!

48. Herbal Healing for Dyspnea: A Natural Recipe for Relief

In our fast-paced lives, it's easy to overlook the signs our bodies give us. For many, dyspnea, or shortness of breath, is a condition that can be both frightening and limiting. It's essential to address the causes of this discomfort, whether they are rooted in anxiety, respiratory issues, or other health concerns. While traditional medical approaches are vital, many individuals also seek natural remedies to complement their treatment plans. Today, we explore an herbal recipe that may help alleviate dyspnea and support overall respiratory health.

Understanding Dyspnea

Dyspnea can be the result of various factors, including allergies, asthma, bronchitis, pneumonia, or heart conditions. It can manifest as a feeling of breathlessness, tightness in the chest, or an increased effort to breathe. Before trying any herbal remedy, it's important to consult with a healthcare professional to understand the underlying causes and ensure a safe approach.

Herbal Healing: Nature's Bounty for Breathing

Several herbs have been traditionally used to support respiratory health and improve breathing. Here's a simple herbal healing recipe that incorporates some of these beneficial ingredients:

Herbal Dyspnea Relief Tea
Ingredients:

- 1 tablespoon dried mullein leaves
- 1 tablespoon dried peppermint
- 1 tablespoon dried thyme
- 1 tablespoon dried marshmallow root
- 4 cups of water
- Honey (optional, to taste)
- Lemon juice (optional, for added flavor)

Instructions:

1. **Combine the Herbs:** In a bowl, mix the dried mullein, peppermint, thyme, and marshmallow root. Each of these herbs contributes unique properties that can promote respiratory health:
   - **Mullein** is known for its expectorant properties and may help soothe the respiratory tract.
   - **Peppermint** offers a refreshing flavor and has menthol, which may help open airways.
   - **Thyme** is rich in antioxidants and can help clear mucus from the lungs.
   - **Marshmallow root** is known for its soothing properties and can help ease irritation in the throat and lungs.
2. **Boil the Water:** In a pot, bring 4 cups of water to a boil.

3. **Steep the Herbs:** Once the water has boiled, remove it from heat and add the herbal mixture. Cover and let it steep for about 10-15 minutes to allow the flavors and beneficial properties to infuse into the water.
4. **Strain the Tea:** After steeping, strain the herbs using a fine mesh strainer or cheesecloth, pouring the liquid into a teapot or a heat-resistant container.
5. **Serve:** Enjoy your herbal tea warm. Add honey for sweetness and lemon juice for a citrusy zing, if desired. Sipping this tea may provide a comforting relief to those experiencing dyspnea.

Additional Tips for Use:

- **Frequency:** You may drink this herbal tea up to three times a day as part of your routine, but listen to your body and adjust as needed.
- **Breathing Exercises:** Companion self-care strategies, such as deep breathing exercises, can enhance the effects of the tea. Practicing slow, diaphragmatic breathing may help calm the body and improve oxygenation.
- **Humidity:** Keeping the environment humid can also alleviate some respiratory discomfort. Consider using a humidifier, especially in dry seasons.

Notes of Caution

While herbal remedies can provide relief, they should not replace medical treatment for chronic conditions. Always consult with a healthcare provider if you experience persistent dyspnea or have underlying health issues. Some herbs may interact with medications, so ensuring a safe approach is paramount.

Nature can provide us with an array of tools for healing, and this herbal remedy for dyspnea highlights the potential benefits of incorporating herbs into our wellness routines. By taking proactive steps towards understanding and addressing our health, we can empower ourselves to breathe easier and live more fully. Embrace the wisdom of nature and nurture your body with this simple herbal tea recipe.

49. Embracing Nature: An Herbal Healing Recipe for Infertility

Infertility can be a challenging journey for many couples, filled with emotional ups and downs. While medical advancements have provided a wealth of options, many people are turning to nature for support in their fertility journeys. Herbal medicine, with its rich tradition and healing properties, offers various remedies that may help enhance fertility. If you're considering incorporating herbal remedies into your routine, here's a gentle yet effective herbal healing recipe to support reproductive health.

Understanding Infertility and Herbal Support

Infertility can stem from various factors, including hormonal imbalances, environmental influences, and lifestyle choices. Herbs have been used for centuries in traditional medicine to support fertility by regulating hormonal balance, improving circulation, and reducing stress—all crucial elements for reproductive health.

An Herbal Tea Recipe for Fertility

This herbal tea blend combines several potent herbs known for their fertility-boosting properties:

Ingredients:

1. **Red Clover Blossoms (1 part)**
   Rich in phytoestrogens, red clover is

believed to help balance hormones and improve overall reproductive health.

2. **Nettle Leaf (1 part)**
   Packed with vitamins and minerals, nettle strengthens the uterus and boosts ovulatory function while providing nourishment to the body.

3. **Raspberry Leaf (1 part)**
   Often used for its tonifying properties, raspberry leaf helps to strengthen the uterine muscles and regulate menstrual cycles.

4. **Maca Root (1 part)** (optional, powdered form)
   Maca is an adaptogen that supports hormonal balance and has been shown to improve fertility in both men and women.

5. **Honey (to taste)** (optional)
   For added sweetness and natural energy.

Instructions:

1. **Prepare the Herbs**: If you're using dried herbs, gently crush them to release their properties. You can mix the equal parts of each herb in a bowl and store them in an airtight container.

2. **Brew the Tea**:
   - Boil 4 cups of water.
   - Add 3 tablespoons of your herbal blend to the boiling water.
   - Lower the heat and let it simmer for about 10-15 minutes.
   - Remove from heat and allow it to steep for an additional 5-10 minutes.

3. **Strain and Serve**: Use a fine mesh strainer or cheesecloth to strain the herbs from the liquid. Pour the tea into your favorite cup and add honey to taste, if desired.
4. **Enjoy**: Drink 1-2 cups of this herbal tea daily. You can also enjoy it chilled as an iced tea during warmer months.

Additional Tips for Enhancing Fertility Naturally

- **Stay Hydrated**: Ensure you're drinking enough water daily, as hydration plays a crucial role in overall health and fertility.
- **Balanced Diet**: Incorporate nutrient-dense foods, such as fresh fruits, vegetables, whole grains, and healthy fats, to support your body's needs.
- **Regular Exercise**: Engage in moderate physical activity to maintain a healthy weight and reduce stress levels.
- **Stress Management**: Consider practices like yoga, meditation, and mindfulness to help manage stress, which can adversely affect fertility.
- **Consultation with a Practitioner**: Before starting any herbal regimen, it's crucial to consult with a healthcare professional or a certified herbalist, especially if you are already on medication or have underlying health conditions.

While the path to fertility can be daunting, turning to herbal remedies can provide gentle support along the way. This herbal tea blend is a nourishing addition to your routine, rich in tradition and potential.

Every individual's body is unique, and what works for one person may not work for another. Therefore, listen to your body, stay informed, and seek guidance from professionals as you explore natural options for enhancing fertility. Celebrate each small step in your journey, and nurture yourself with love, patience, and the healing power of nature.

50. Herbal Healing for Endometriosis: A Holistic Approach

Endometriosis is a challenging condition that affects millions of women worldwide, often causing debilitating pain, heavy menstrual bleeding, and a host of other symptoms. While traditional treatments like hormonal therapies and surgeries are common, many women are seeking natural alternatives to alleviate their symptoms and promote healing. In the information below, we'll study an herbal healing recipe that may help manage the symptoms of endometriosis.

Understanding Endometriosis

Endometriosis occurs when tissue similar to the lining of the uterus (the endometrium) grows outside the uterus, often leading to inflammation, pain, and scar tissue formation. Symptoms can vary widely, and while there's no cure, many women find relief through lifestyle changes, dietary adjustments, and natural remedies.

The Power of Herbs

Herbs have been used for centuries in various cultures to manage women's health issues, including menstrual disorders and reproductive health concerns. They can help to reduce inflammation, regulate hormones, relieve pain, and support overall wellness.

An Herbal Healing Recipe: Endo Relief Tea

Here's a simple herbal tea recipe that may help alleviate some symptoms of endometriosis. This blend combines anti-inflammatory, hormone-regulating, and soothing herbs, making it both beneficial and delicious.

Ingredients:

1. **2 tablespoons of Red Clover (Trifolium pratense)**
   - Known for its phytoestrogens, red clover can help balance hormones and reduce the severity of menstrual discomfort.
2. **1 tablespoon of Ginger root (Zingiber officinale)**
   - Ginger is a powerful anti-inflammatory that can help relieve pain and cramping.
3. **1 tablespoon of Chamomile flowers (Matricaria chamomilla)**
   - Chamomile is gently calming and can help reduce stress and anxiety, promoting relaxation and pain relief.
4. **1 tablespoon of Turmeric root (Curcuma longa)**
   - Turmeric contains curcumin, a potent anti-inflammatory compound that may help reduce pelvic pain.
5. **1 tablespoon of Dong Quai (Angelica sinensis)** (optional)

o Known as a female tonic in Traditional Chinese Medicine, Dong Quai may help regulate the menstrual cycle and support overall reproductive health.

6. **4 cups of water**
7. **Honey or lemon (optional for taste)**

Instructions:

1. **Prepare the herbs**: Measure out the herbs and mix them in a small bowl.
2. **Boil the water**: Bring 4 cups of water to a boil in a pot.
3. **Steep the herbs**: Once the water reaches a boil, remove it from the heat and add the mixed herbs. Cover the pot to let the herbs steep for about 15-20 minutes.
4. **Strain and serve**: After steeping, strain the tea into a teapot or teacup. You can add honey or lemon for taste if desired.
5. **Enjoy**: Drink this tea up to three times a day, particularly during your menstrual cycle or when you experience discomfort.

Tips for Enhancement

- **Dietary Considerations**: Pair this tea with an anti-inflammatory diet rich in whole foods, fruits, vegetables, nuts, seeds, and lean proteins. Avoiding processed foods, excessive sugar, and dairy may also help reduce inflammation.
- **Stay Hydrated**: Drink plenty of water throughout the day to support your body and reduce bloating.

- **Consult a Healthcare Professional**: Always consult with a healthcare provider, especially if you are taking other medications or have underlying health conditions. Herbs can interact with medications, and it's important to ensure that a holistic approach fits your individual health needs.

Final Thoughts

Endometriosis can be a complex and painful condition, but with the right support and strategies, it is possible to find relief. This herbal healing tea is just one approach among many holistic interventions that may help manage symptoms and promote well-being. Always listen to your body. Believing in a natural, herbal approach can empower you to take control of your health, even during challenging times.

Cheers to your journey toward healing and balance!

51. Herbal Healing for Prostate Health: A Home Remedy Recipe

As more individuals turn to natural remedies to support their health, herbal treatments have gained acclaim for their potential benefits, especially for prostate health. The prostate is a small gland, but it plays a significant role in male reproductive health. Common issues associated with the prostate include benign prostatic hyperplasia (BPH), prostatitis, and in more severe cases, prostate cancer. While professional medical advice is essential for diagnosis and treatment, herbal remedies can complement a healthcare plan and promote overall well-being.

This recipe incorporates a blend of powerful herbs known for their beneficial properties concerning the prostate.

Key Ingredients

1. Saw Palmetto (Serenoa repens): Saw palmetto is one of the most studied herbs for prostate health. It is believed to inhibit the conversion of testosterone to dihydrotestosterone (DHT), a hormone linked to prostate enlargement.

2. Nettle Root (Urtica dioica): Nettle root is traditionally used for urinary tract issues and is thought to help relieve symptoms associated with BPH, such as frequent urination and discomfort.

3. Pygeum (Prunus africana): Extract from the bark of the African plum tree, pygeum is another herb reputed to support prostate health, promoting better urinary function.

4. Turmeric (Curcuma longa): Turmeric contains curcumin, a powerful anti-inflammatory and antioxidant compound, which may help reduce inflammation in the prostate and surrounding tissues.

5. Green Tea (Camellia sinensis): Rich in antioxidants, particularly catechins, green tea may help protect prostate health and potentially lower the risk of prostate issues.

Relaxing Herbal Tea Recipe for Prostate Health

This invigorating herbal tea combines the aforementioned ingredients into a delicious and health-boosting beverage.

Ingredients:

- 1 tsp dried saw palmetto berries (or 1 tsp saw palmetto extract)
- 1 tsp dried nettle root
- 1 tsp dried pygeum bark (or pygeum extract)
- 1/2 tsp turmeric powder (or fresh turmeric root, grated)
- 1 green tea bag (or 1 tsp loose green tea)
- 4 cups of water
- Honey or lemon (optional, for taste)

Instructions:

1. **Combine the Ingredients:** In a saucepan, add the dried saw palmetto, nettle root, pygeum bark, turmeric powder, and water. If using extracts, you can add them later in the brewing process for better effectiveness.
2. **Boil the Mixture:** Bring the mixture to a gentle boil over medium heat. Once boiling, reduce to low heat and let it simmer for about 20 minutes. This allows the nutrients and beneficial compounds to infuse into the water.
3. **Add the Green Tea:** After 20 minutes, remove the saucepan from heat and add the green tea bag. Let it steep for an additional 5-7 minutes, depending on how strong you prefer your tea.
4. **Strain and Serve:** Use a fine mesh strainer to pour the tea into a teapot or individual cups, discarding the herbs. If desired, sweeten with honey or add a squeeze of lemon for an extra burst of flavor.
5. **Enjoy:** Sip this herbal tea 1-2 times a day to support your prostate health, combining it with a balanced diet, regular exercise, and hydration.

Additional Tips for Prostate Health

- **Maintain a Healthy Diet:** Incorporating foods rich in omega-3 fatty acids, fruits, and vegetables can provide additional support.

- **Stay Hydrated:** Aim for at least 8 glasses of water a day, as hydration helps facilitate urinary function.
- **Exercise Regularly:** Physical activity is crucial for overall health and can help alleviate symptoms associated with prostate issues.
- **Consult with a Healthcare Professional:** Always get advice from a qualified healthcare provider, especially if you have pre-existing conditions or are taking medications.

Herbal remedies can be a valuable part of your journey toward better prostate health. This herbal tea recipe harnesses the power of nature's ingredients, making it a simple yet effective addition to your daily wellness routine. Remember, while herbs can provide support, they are best used in conjunction with conventional medical care. Always prioritize your health by consulting with professionals who can guide you in your pursuit of wellness.

Cheers to your health!

52. Herbal Healing Recipe for Obesity: A Natural Approach to Wellness

In a world where quick fixes and fad diets dominate the weight loss conversation, it's essential to return to the roots of natural healing. For those struggling with obesity, adopting a holistic approach that emphasizes whole foods and herbal remedies can not only aid weight loss but also promote overall health and well-being.

Understanding Obesity

Before we delve into our herbal recipe, it's important to understand what obesity is. Obesity is a complex health condition characterized by an excessive accumulation of body fat. It increases the risk of various chronic diseases, including heart disease, diabetes, and certain cancers. Managing obesity involves a multifaceted approach, including dietary changes, physical activity, and, potentially, herbal support.

The Role of Herbs in Weight Management

Herbs and natural remedies have been utilized for centuries in various cultures to promote health and healing. Many herbs possess properties that can aid weight loss by:

1. **Boosting Metabolism**: Certain herbs can increase metabolic rate, helping the body burn more calories.
2. **Suppressing Appetite**: Some herbs can help control cravings and promote a feeling of fullness.
3. **Balancing Blood Sugar**: Herbs that help regulate blood sugar can prevent spikes and crashes that lead to unhealthy snacking.

Herbal Healing Recipe: Detoxifying Green Tea Elixir

This simple yet potent herbal recipe combines powerful ingredients known for their weight management properties. It's refreshing, easy to prepare, and can be consumed daily for optimal benefits.

Ingredients

- **2 cups of filtered water**
- **1 tablespoon of green tea leaves (or 1 green tea bag)**
- **1 teaspoon of dried dandelion root**
- **1 teaspoon of dried hibiscus flowers**
- **½ teaspoon of fresh mint leaves (or ½ teaspoon of dried mint)**
- **1-2 teaspoons of raw honey (optional)**
- **Juice of half a lemon**

Instructions

1. **Boil Water**: In a saucepan, bring 2 cups of filtered water to a boil.

2. **Add Herbs**: Once boiling, remove the saucepan from heat. Add the green tea leaves, dandelion root, hibiscus flowers, and mint leaves.
3. **Steep**: Cover and steep the mixture for about 10 minutes. This allows the herbs to infuse their beneficial properties into the water.
4. **Strain**: After steeping, strain the tea into a mug, discarding the solid herbs.
5. **Add Flavor**: Stir in the honey (if using) and the juice of half a lemon for a delicious tang.
6. **Enjoy**: Sip the tea warm or let it cool and enjoy over ice as a refreshing cold beverage.

Health Benefits of the Ingredients

- **Green Tea**: Rich in antioxidants and catechins, green tea is well-known for its ability to boost metabolism and enhance fat burning.
- **Dandelion Root**: This herb acts as a natural diuretic, promoting detoxification and reducing water retention. It also supports liver health.
- **Hibiscus Flowers**: Hibiscus tea has been linked to lower blood pressure and may also assist in reducing body fat and waist size.
- **Mint**: Mint can help soothe the digestive system and curb appetite, making it easier to stick to healthy eating habits.
- **Lemon**: High in vitamin C and antioxidants, lemon supports metabolism and detoxification efforts.

Incorporating Herbal Healing into Your Lifestyle

While this herbal elixir can be a valuable addition to your daily routine, remember that managing obesity is a holistic endeavor. Here are some tips to incorporate alongside your herbal remedy:

1. **Balanced Diet**: Focus on whole foods, including fruits, vegetables, lean proteins, and whole grains.
2. **Regular Exercise**: Aim for at least 150 minutes of moderate-intensity exercise each week, such as brisk walking, cycling, or swimming.
3. **Mindful Eating**: Pay attention to portion sizes and practice mindful eating to help control cravings and enhance satisfaction.
4. **Stay Hydrated**: Drink plenty of water throughout the day to support metabolism and reduce hunger.
5. **Consult Health Professionals**: Always consult with a healthcare provider or herbalist before starting any new herbal remedy, especially if you have underlying health conditions or are on medication.

Herbal remedies can be a powerful tool in the journey toward weight management. The Detoxifying Green Tea Elixir is not only a delicious beverage but also a natural way to support your body in achieving its weight loss goals. Remember, consistency is key, and combining this herbal approach with a healthy lifestyle can lead to lasting results. Be open to this natural journey to wellness, and take a step forward in transforming your health one sip at a time!

53. Herbal Healing Recipe for Sciatica: Nature's Remedy for Nerve Pain

Living with sciatica can be a debilitating experience. Characterized by pain radiating from the lower back down through the legs, sciatica often occurs due to nerve compression, herniated discs, or other underlying issues. While conventional treatments like physical therapy and medications are common, many people are increasingly turning to herbal remedies to find relief.

Understanding Sciatica

Before we dive into the herbal recipe, let's briefly discuss what sciatica is. The sciatic nerve is the longest nerve in the body, running from the lower back down through the buttocks and into each leg. When this nerve is compressed or irritated, it can lead to pain, numbness, or weakness in the lower back, buttocks, and legs.

Typical causes of sciatica include:

- Herniated or slipped discs
- Spinal stenosis
- Spondylolisthesis
- Piriformis syndrome

Herbal Healing Recipe for Sciatica

Ingredients

1. **Turmeric (Curcuma longa)** - 1 tablespoon of dried powder
   - o **Benefits:** Known for its anti-inflammatory properties, turmeric contains curcumin, which can help reduce pain and inflammation associated with sciatica.
2. **Ginger (Zingiber officinale)** - 1 tablespoon of grated fresh ginger or 1 teaspoon of dried ginger powder
   - o **Benefits:** Ginger also possesses anti-inflammatory properties and can help relieve muscle tension.
3. **Willow Bark (Salix spp.)** - 1 teaspoon of dried bark
   - o **Benefits:** Often referred to as nature's aspirin, willow bark contains salicin, which has analgesic properties.
4. **Cayenne Pepper (Capsicum annuum)** - 1/2 teaspoon of powdered cayenne
   - o **Benefits:** Capsaicin in cayenne pepper can provide pain relief by blocking pain signals to the brain.
5. **Apple Cider Vinegar** - 1 tablespoon
   - o **Benefits:** Known for its alkalizing properties and potential for reducing inflammation.
6. **Warm Water** - 1 cup
7. **Honey** (optional) - 1 teaspoon

Instructions

1. **Prepare the Herbal Infusion:**
   o In a saucepan, bring one cup of warm water to a gentle simmer.
   o Add the turmeric, ginger, willow bark, and cayenne pepper to the water. Stir well to combine.
2. **Simmer:**
   o Allow the mixture to simmer for about 10-15 minutes. This helps extract the beneficial compounds from the herbs.
3. **Strain:**
   o After simmering, remove the saucepan from heat and strain the mixture using a fine mesh strainer or a cheesecloth into a mug, discarding the solid herbs.
4. **Add Apple Cider Vinegar and Honey:**
   o Stir in the apple cider vinegar. If desired, sweeten the infusion with honey for taste.
5. **Serve:**
   o Enjoy the herbal infusion warm. You can drink this once or twice daily for relief.

Additional Tips for Healing

- **Stay Hydrated:** Drink plenty of water throughout the day to help with overall inflammation.
- **Gentle Stretching:** Incorporate gentle stretching exercises into your daily routine to help alleviate pressure on the sciatic nerve.

- **Hot/Cold Compresses:** Use hot compresses on the lower back to reduce pain or cold packs to numb inflammation.
- **Consult a Professional:** Always consult a healthcare provider before starting any new herbal regimen, especially if you have underlying health conditions or are on medication.

Final Thoughts

While the herbal recipe provided is a natural way to address sciatica symptoms, it's essential to remember that every individual's body responds differently to herbs. Results may vary, and combining herbal remedies with a holistic approach—including proper physical therapy, diet, and lifestyle modifications—often yields the best outcomes.

Embrace the healing power of nature, and don't hesitate to reach out to a qualified herbalist or healthcare provider for personalized guidance. Here's to your journey toward relief and recovery!

54. Embrace Spring with Herbal Healing: A Soothing Recipe for Seasonal Allergies

As the flowers bloom and the leaves unfurl, many of us welcome the joys of spring. However, for millions, the season comes with a familiar foe: seasonal allergies. Pollen, grass, and mold can ignite sneezing, itchy eyes, and congestion, turning a beautiful day into a struggle for breath. But fear not! Nature offers an array of soothing remedies to help alleviate allergy symptoms. Below, we'll explore an herbal healing recipe that you can easily make at home to soothe your seasonal allergy woes.

Understanding Seasonal Allergies

Seasonal allergies, also known as hay fever or allergic rhinitis, occur when your immune system overreacts to allergens in the environment, primarily pollen from trees, grasses, and weeds. Symptoms can vary in severity and typically include:

- Sneezing and runny nose
- Itchy and watery eyes
- Congestion
- Fatigue
- Scratchy throat

While over-the-counter medications might provide temporary relief, many people are turning to natural remedies for a more holistic approach. Herbs have been used for centuries to relieve allergy symptoms, and with a little knowledge, you can harness their power right from your kitchen.

An Herbal Healing Recipe: Allergy Relief Tea

This delicious herbal tea blend combines powerful, natural ingredients that have been traditionally used to combat the symptoms of seasonal allergies. With anti-inflammatory, antihistamine, and immune-boosting properties, this tea can be a soothing addition to your daily routine.

Ingredients

- **1 teaspoon dried nettle leaf**: Nettle has natural antihistamine properties and can help reduce nasal inflammation.
- **1 teaspoon dried chamomile flowers**: Chamomile is known for its soothing effects and can help ease irritation in the respiratory system.
- **1 teaspoon dried peppermint leaves**: Peppermint aids in opening the airways and can help relieve nasal congestion.
- **1 teaspoon dried elderflower**: Elderflower has been used to soothe upper respiratory tract infections and can also stimulate the immune system.

- **1 tablespoon raw honey (optional)**: Honey can add sweetness while also providing its own anti-inflammatory benefits.
- **2 cups hot water**
- **Juice of half a lemon (optional)**: Lemon adds a refreshing zing and vitamin C, which supports the immune system.

Instructions

1. **Combine the Herbs**: In a small bowl, mix the dried nettle, chamomile, peppermint, and elderflower.
2. **Boil Water**: Heat 2 cups of water to a rolling boil.
3. **Infuse the Tea**: Place the herbal mix in a teapot or a large mug and pour the hot water over the herbs. Cover and let steep for about 10 minutes. This allows the medicinal properties of the herbs to infuse into the water.
4. **Strain and Serve**: After steeping, strain the tea into another mug to remove the herbs. If desired, stir in the raw honey for sweetness and the lemon juice for added flavor.
5. **Sip and Soothe**: Enjoy your herbal tea warm, and sip it throughout the day whenever you feel the symptoms of allergies creeping in.

Tips for Maximizing Effectiveness

- **Consistency is Key**: For best results, drink this tea daily during allergy season.

- **Stay Hydrated**: Complement your herbal tea with plenty of water to stay hydrated and help your body flush out allergens.
- **Maintain a Clean Environment**: Keep windows and doors closed during high pollen counts, and consider using air purifiers to reduce allergens in your home.

When to See a Doctor

While herbal remedies can be incredibly beneficial, it's essential to consult a healthcare professional if your symptoms persist or worsen. Severe allergic reactions may require prompt medical attention.

Seasonal allergies can put a damper on the joy of spring, but Mother Nature has given us helpful tools to combat these symptoms. This simple herbal tea recipe offers a natural, calming solution that's easy to make and delightful to consume. Believe in the beauty of the season with this soothing remedy, and may your spring be filled with fresh blossoms, sunshine, and clear skies!

55. Herbal Healing for Hepatitis: A Natural Approach to Liver Health

Hepatitis, an inflammation of the liver often caused by viral infections, alcoholism, or autoimmune diseases, poses significant health challenges. While it's crucial to seek professional medical advice and treatment when dealing with hepatitis, certain herbal remedies may complement conventional therapies and support liver health.

Understanding Hepatitis

Hepatitis can be categorized into several types, including Hepatitis A, B, C, D, and E, each with different causes and modes of transmission. Symptoms can vary but often include fatigue, jaundice, abdominal pain, and loss of appetite. For those struggling with liver health, it's essential to adopt a balanced diet, engage in regular physical activity, and consider holistic remedies, including herbs that have been used traditionally for liver support.

Herbal Ingredients for Liver Health

Before we dive into the recipe, let's look at some herbs that have been credited with liver restorative properties:

1. **Milk Thistle (Silybum marianum)**: Known for its active compound silibinin, milk thistle protects the liver from toxins and promotes cell regeneration.
2. **Dandelion Root (Taraxacum officinale)**: This common weed is renowned for its detoxifying properties and is traditionally used to stimulate bile flow, aiding digestion and liver function.
3. **Turmeric (Curcuma longa)**: Curcumin, the active component in turmeric, is a potent anti-inflammatory and antioxidant that supports liver detoxification processes.
4. **Artichoke (Cynara scolymus)**: Used for centuries, artichoke extract is believed to improve liver function and enhance bile production.
5. **Lemon Balm (Melissa officinalis)**: This herb has calming properties and aids digestion, making it a soothing addition for liver health.

Herbal Healing Recipe for Liver Support

Ingredients:

- 1 teaspoon of dried Milk Thistle seeds
- 1 teaspoon of Dandelion root
- 1 teaspoon of Turmeric powder
- 1 teaspoon of dried Artichoke leaves
- 1 teaspoon of dried Lemon Balm
- 4 cups of water
- Honey (optional, for taste)

Instructions:

1. **Prepare Your Herbs**: Measure out each herb and combine them in a bowl. If you have whole Milk Thistle seeds or Dandelion root, you may wish to lightly crush them to release their beneficial oils.
2. **Boil the Water**: In a saucepan, bring 4 cups of water to a boil.
3. **Add the Herbs**: Once the water is boiling, add your mixed herbs. Reduce the heat to low, cover, and let it simmer for about 20 minutes. This process allows the herbs to release their beneficial compounds into the water.
4. **Strain the Tea**: After simmering, remove the saucepan from the heat and strain the mixture into a teapot or container. Discard the herbs.
5. **Flavor (Optional)**: If you find the taste too earthy or bitter, sweeten your tea with a little honey to suit your preference.
6. **Serve and Enjoy**: Drink this herbal infusion 1 to 2 times daily. Be sure to enjoy it fresh, as the active compounds are best when consumed shortly after preparation.

Additional Lifestyle Tips

While herbal remedies can play a supportive role in liver health, here are a few additional lifestyle changes to consider:

- **Stay Hydrated**: Drinking plenty of water helps flush toxins from your body.
- **Eat a Balanced Diet**: Focus on whole foods, including fruits, vegetables, whole

grains, and lean proteins. Avoid processed
foods and excessive sugar.
* **Limit Alcohol Intake**: Alcohol can
exacerbate liver damage, so moderating or
abstaining altogether is advisable.
* **Exercise Regularly**: Engaging in regular
physical activity promotes overall health
and helps maintain a healthy weight.

Consult with a Professional

Before embarking on any herbal remedy, it's
essential to consult with a healthcare
professional, especially if you have a pre-existing
health condition or are taking prescription
medications. They can provide personalized
recommendations and ensure safe and effective
treatment options tailored to your needs.

While herbs alone are not a cure for hepatitis,
they can serve as a valuable support system for
liver health when used in conjunction with
medical treatment. This herbal healing recipe
brings together traditional wisdom and the power
of nature, offering a refreshing way to nourish
and support your liver. Take care of your health,
embrace natural remedies, and prioritize self-
care—your liver will thank you!

56. Herbal Healing for Respiratory Distress: A Natural Recipe

As the seasons shift and our exposure to environmental irritants fluctuate, many of us might experience respiratory distress. Whether due to allergies, colds, or irritants in our environment, finding natural ways to support our respiratory health can be invaluable.

Understanding Respiratory Distress

Respiratory distress can manifest as coughing, wheezing, difficulty breathing, or a feeling of tightness in the chest. Common causes include respiratory infections, allergies, asthma, or pollutants in the air. While it's essential to consult a healthcare provider for persistent or severe symptoms, many have turned to nature for support, seeking out herbal remedies that can provide relief.

Herbal Ingredients

The following herbs are known for their potential benefits in supporting respiratory function:

1. **Thyme**: Known for its antimicrobial properties, thyme can help clear mucus and soothe the throat.

2. **Peppermint**: With its menthol content, peppermint can ease congestion and open up the airways.
3. **Eucalyptus**: Often used in steam inhalation, eucalyptus can help to relieve cough and promote easier breathing.
4. **Chamomile**: This calming herb can help soothe inflammation and promote relaxation during bouts of respiratory distress.
5. **Ginger**: Not only does ginger have anti-inflammatory properties, but it can also help the body fight off infections.

Herbal Healing Recipe for Respiratory Distress

Ingredients:

- 1 teaspoon dried thyme
- 1 teaspoon dried peppermint
- 1 teaspoon dried eucalyptus leaves
- 1 teaspoon dried chamomile flowers
- 1 teaspoon fresh ginger root (or ½ teaspoon dried ginger)
- 2 cups water
- Honey (optional, to taste)
- Lemon juice (optional, to taste)

Instructions:

1. **Prepare the Ingredients**: Measure out the dried herbs and fresh ginger root. If using fresh ginger, peel and slice it thinly to maximize flavor and medicinal properties.

2. **Boil the Water**: In a saucepan, bring two cups of water to a gentle boil.
3. **Add the Herbs**: Once the water is boiling, reduce the heat to a simmer. Add thyme, peppermint, eucalyptus, chamomile, and ginger to the water.
4. **Steep the Mixture**: Allow the herbs to steep for 10-15 minutes. This will help extract their beneficial properties.
5. **Strain and Serve**: After steeping, strain the mixture through a fine-mesh sieve or cheesecloth into a mug.
6. **Add Sweetness and Flavor**: If desired, add honey and lemon juice to taste. Honey not only sweetens the tea but also has soothing properties, while lemon can provide a dose of vitamin C.
7. **Enjoy**: Sip the herbal tea slowly, taking a moment to breathe in the steam as you enjoy the warm, soothing beverage.

Additional Tips

- **Steam Inhalation**: After making the tea, consider using the leftover herbal blend for steam inhalation. Simply pour it into a bowl, cover your head with a towel, and inhale the steam for added respiratory relief.
- **Humidifier**: If your environment is dry, consider using a humidifier to keep the air moist, as this can help ease respiratory discomfort.

- **Stay Hydrated**: Drink plenty of fluids to help thin mucus and keep your airways clear.

Caution

While this herbal remedy can offer relief for mild respiratory distress, it is crucial to consult a healthcare provider if symptoms persist, worsen, or if you have underlying health conditions like asthma or chronic lung disease. Always check for potential allergies to any of the ingredients before consuming.

Embracing nature's pharmacy can provide soothing relief in times of respiratory distress. This herbal tea recipe combines gentle, effective ingredients that work together to support your respiratory health. So the next time you find yourself struggling to breathe freely, reach for this herbal remedy rather than relying solely on conventional treatments. Your lungs—and your overall well-being—will thank you!

57. Harnessing the Power of Nature: An Herbal Healing Recipe for Stroke Recovery

Stroke is a major health concern that can significantly impact the quality of life. With millions affected worldwide, the road to recovery can often feel daunting. While conventional medicine plays a crucial role in treatment, many individuals seek complementary therapies to support their healing journey. One such option is herbal medicine, which has been used for centuries to promote recovery and overall wellness.

In this section below, we'll explore an herbal healing recipe specifically designed to support stroke recovery and share tips on integrating these herbs into your daily routine.

Understanding Stroke and Its Aftermath

A stroke occurs when the blood supply to a part of the brain is interrupted, leading to cell death and neurological damage. This can result in physical disabilities, cognitive impairments, and emotional challenges. The path to recovery often involves physical therapy, speech therapy, and sometimes medications to prevent further strokes.

However, herbal remedies can serve as valuable allies in this process. Herbs can promote circulation, support cognitive function, and aid in emotional healing. Always consult with a healthcare provider before incorporating any herbal remedies, especially following a medical condition like a stroke.

Herbal Healing Recipe: "Recovery Tonic Blend"

This herbal blend combines several powerful ingredients known for their healing properties.

Ingredients:
- **Ginkgo Biloba (1 tablespoon):** Known for its ability to improve blood flow and enhance cognitive function, ginkgo biloba can help support brain health post-stroke.
- **Turmeric (1 tablespoon):** This golden spice contains curcumin, a potent anti-inflammatory and antioxidant that may aid in brain recovery and reduce inflammation.
- **Bacopa Monnieri (1 tablespoon):** Often used in traditional Ayurvedic medicine, bacopa is believed to enhance memory and cognitive function.
- **Lemon Balm (1 tablespoon):** This calming herb can help reduce anxiety and improve mood, fostering a positive mindset during recovery.
- **Honey (to taste):** A natural sweetener known for its soothing properties and ability to support overall health.

Instructions:

1. **Preparation**: In a small pot, bring 2 cups of water to a boil.
2. **Mix the Herbs**: Once boiling, reduce the heat and add the ginkgo biloba, turmeric, bacopa, and lemon balm.
3. **Simmer**: Allow the mixture to simmer for about 10-15 minutes. This process extracts the beneficial compounds from the herbs.
4. **Strain**: After simmering, carefully strain the herbs using a fine mesh strainer or cheesecloth into a clean container.
5. **Sweeten**: Add honey to taste while the tonic is still warm, ensuring it dissolves fully.
6. **Consume**: Allow the tonic to cool slightly before consuming. Drink one cup daily, ideally in the morning, to set a positive tone for your day.

Additional Tips for Integrating Herbal Remedies

1. **Consistency is Key**: Like any healing approach, consistency is vital. Incorporate the Recovery Tonic Blend into your daily routine, but remember that herbal remedies are not replacements for medical treatments.
2. **Combine with a Healthy Diet**: Pair this tonic with a balanced diet rich in fruits, vegetables, whole grains, and healthy fats. Foods high in omega-3 fatty acids, such as fish and flaxseed, can be particularly beneficial for brain health.

3. **Stay Hydrated**: Drinking plenty of water is essential for overall recovery and helps to transport the beneficial compounds from your herbs.
4. **Engage in Mild Exercise**: If approved by your healthcare provider, gentle activities like walking or yoga can support your recovery and enhance the benefits of herbal remedies.
5. **Mind Your Mental Health**: Emotional well-being is a significant aspect of stroke recovery. Integrate mindfulness practices such as meditation, deep breathing exercises, or gentle movement to foster mental clarity and reduce stress.

Listening to Your Body

Every individual's recovery journey is unique, and herbal remedies can work differently for everyone. Be sure to listen to your body and observe how you feel after incorporating the Recovery Tonic Blend and other herbal treatments. If you notice any adverse effects, discontinue use and consult with a healthcare professional.

While recovery from a stroke can be a challenging journey, incorporating herbal remedies like the Recovery Tonic Blend can provide support and promote healing. With the right blend of herbal wisdom, a healthy lifestyle, and conventional medical care, you can pave the way to a brighter, healthier future. Remember to consult with your healthcare provider before starting any new treatment and celebrate each step you take towards recovery.

Nature has a remarkable way of supporting us, so why not embrace its healing power?

58. Herbal Healing Recipe for Candida: Embrace Nature's Remedies

Candida overgrowth can be an uncomfortable and frustrating condition. Often manifesting as yeast infections, digestive issues, or skin irritations, it thrives in overly sugary and processed environments, making it crucial to find a natural approach to rebalance your system. The good news is that various herbs can help combat candida while promoting overall health.

Understanding Candida Overgrowth

Candida is a type of yeast that naturally exists in our bodies, primarily in the gut. When our internal environment is thrown off balance, candida can multiply rapidly, leading to various symptoms, including:

- Fatigue
- Digestive disturbances (bloating, gas, constipation)
- Skin issues (rashes, eczema)
- Cravings for sugar

To combat candida, it's essential to create an unwelcoming environment for the yeast. This typically involves reducing sugar intake and incorporating antifungal and supportive herbs into your diet.

Herbal Ingredients to Heal Candida

Before we dive into the recipe, let's highlight some key herbs known for their antifungal and healing properties:

1. **Garlic**: This potent herb contains allicin, which has been shown to possess antifungal properties, making it effective against candida. Plus, garlic boosts the immune system!
2. **Oregano Oil**: Known for its powerful antibacterial and antifungal effects, oregano oil can help reduce candida overgrowth.
3. **Coconut Oil**: Rich in medium-chain fatty acids, coconut oil has antifungal properties and can disrupt the cell membranes of candida.
4. **Ginger**: With its anti-inflammatory and digestive benefits, ginger can help soothe the gut while supporting detoxification and digestion.
5. **Turmeric**: Curcumin, the active compound in turmeric, has strong antifungal, anti-inflammatory, and antioxidant properties. It's excellent for overall health and immunity.
6. **Cinnamon**: Known for its ability to regulate blood sugar levels, cinnamon may help keep blood sugar levels stable and reduce the risk of candida overgrowth.

Herbal Healing Recipe: Anti-Candida Tea

This flavorful tea combines several potent herbs to create a soothing, antifungal drink that can help restore balance in your body. Pair it with a healthy diet low in sugar and refined carbohydrates to maximize results.

Ingredients

- 1 teaspoon dried oregano
- 1 teaspoon dried ginger
- 1 teaspoon dried turmeric
- ½ teaspoon ground cinnamon (or 1 cinnamon stick)
- 2 cloves of garlic, crushed
- 2 cups water
- 1-2 teaspoons honey (optional; use sparingly)

Instructions

1. **Boil Water**: In a pot, bring 2 cups of water to a boil.
2. **Add Herbs**: Once boiling, add the dried oregano, ginger, turmeric, cinnamon, and crushed garlic.
3. **Simmer**: Reduce the heat to low and let it simmer for about 10-15 minutes. This allows the herbs to infuse their potent properties into the water.
4. **Strain**: After simmering, strain the tea into a cup to remove the solids.
5. **Sweeten (Optional)**: If desired, add honey for sweetness. Remember, consult with your healthcare provider regarding honey's sugar content if you're managing candida.

6. **Sip and Enjoy**: Enjoy this tea 1-2 times daily as part of your wellness routine.

Additional Tips for Managing Candida

While the herbal tea will support your efforts against candida, consider these additional lifestyle and dietary changes:

- **Limit Sugar and Carbs**: Reduce intake of refined sugars and carbohydrates that can feed candida.
- **Stay Hydrated**: Drink plenty of water to help flush out toxins.
- **Consume Probiotics**: Include fermented foods like yogurt, sauerkraut, and kefir to help restore healthy gut flora.
- **Eat a Balanced Diet**: Focus on whole foods, plenty of vegetables, and healthy fats while avoiding processed foods.

Managing candida overgrowth requires a multi-faceted approach that encompasses diet, lifestyle, and herbal remedies. The herbal tea recipe shared above highlights the potential benefits of nature's ingredients in fighting candida. Always remember to consult with a healthcare professional before significantly altering your diet or trying new herbal remedies, especially if you have underlying health conditions.

Learn the power of herbs, nurture your body, and take the first steps towards healing your candida issues naturally!

59. Harnessing Nature: An Herbal Healing Recipe for Tourette Syndrome

Tourette Syndrome (TS) is a neurological condition characterized by repetitive, involuntary movements and vocalizations known as tics. While it's often diagnosed in childhood, it can persist into adulthood. The complexity of TS lies not only in managing its physical symptoms but also in addressing the emotional and psychological challenges that often accompany it. While conventional treatments like behavioral therapy and medication are common, some individuals look towards herbal remedies as complementary approaches to managing their symptoms.

Here we'll explore an herbal healing recipe that may help alleviate symptoms associated with Tourette Syndrome, combined with lifestyle approaches grounded in mindfulness and self-care.

Understanding the Role of Herbs

Herbal medicine offers a holistic approach to health, emphasizing the interconnection between body and mind. Certain herbs are believed to have properties that could help reduce anxiety, improve mood, and promote a sense of calm — factors that can be beneficial for those with TS.

An Herbal Healing Recipe for Tourette Syndrome

This herbal blend combines anxiety-reducing and calming ingredients that may help soothe the nervous system. However, always consult with a healthcare professional before trying new treatments, especially if you're on medication.

Ingredients:

1. **Lemon Balm (Melissa officinalis)** – 1 part
   - Known for its calming properties, lemon balm can help reduce stress and promote relaxation.
2. **Lavender (Lavandula)** – 1 part
   - Lavender is renowned for its soothing scent and has been shown to have anxiolytic effects, which can help alleviate anxiety and restlessness.
3. **Chamomile (Matricaria chamomilla)** – 1 part
   - Chamomile is well-known for its calming properties and can promote relaxation and sleep.
4. **Passionflower (Passiflora incarnata)** – 1 part
   - This herb has been used traditionally as a mild sedative and has shown promise in reducing anxiety and promoting a sense of well-being.
5. **Hawthorn Berry (Crataegus)** – 1 part
   - Hawthorn is often used in herbal medicine to support heart health and circulation, contributing to overall emotional well-being.

Preparation:

1. **Mix the Herbs**: Combine equal parts of lemon balm, lavender, chamomile, passionflower, and hawthorn berry in a clean, dry jar. Store it in a cool, dark place.
2. **Make an Infusion**: To prepare an herbal infusion, boil 1 cup of water and pour it over 1 tablespoon of the herbal blend. Allow it to steep for about 10-15 minutes.
3. **Strain and Serve**: After steeping, strain the mixture into a cup. You may add honey or lemon for flavor if desired.
4. **Frequency**: Enjoy this tea once to twice daily, particularly during times of heightened stress or anxiety.

Integrating Mindfulness and Lifestyle Changes

While herbal remedies can provide supportive care, lifestyle adjustments play a crucial role in managing Tourette Syndrome. Here are a few suggestions:

1. **Mindfulness Practices**: Engage in mindfulness techniques such as meditation, yoga, or deep breathing exercises. These practices can help center the mind and reduce anxiety.
2. **Regular Exercise**: Physical activity is a fantastic way to reduce stress and improve mood. Aim for at least 30 minutes of moderate exercise most days of the week.
3. **Balanced Diet**: A nutrient-rich diet can positively influence your overall well-being. Focus on whole foods, including fruits,

vegetables, whole grains, lean proteins, and healthy fats.

4. **Adequate Sleep**: Quality sleep is essential for managing stress and maintaining a balanced mood. Establish a bedtime routine that promotes relaxation.
5. **Social Support**: Surround yourself with supportive friends and family. Connecting with others who understand your experiences can be incredibly therapeutic.

While Tourette Syndrome can be challenging, approaching it with a holistic mindset allows individuals to navigate their symptoms more effectively. Incorporating herbal remedies like the one above, combined with mindful living, can empower those dealing with TS to cultivate a sense of balance and well-being. Always remember, it's essential to consult with healthcare providers before starting any new treatments or remedies. Nature provides many tools, but the journey to healing is personal, and support is key.

Embrace the process, and may you find peace and comfort in the herbs that nature has to offer!

60. Herbal Healing for Osteoporosis: A Recipe to Support Bone Health

Osteoporosis, often known as the "silent disease," affects millions of people worldwide, leading to an increased risk of fractures and falls due to weakened bones. With this condition primarily affecting older adults, it's essential to adopt a multifaceted approach that includes proper nutrition, exercise, and, where appropriate, herbal remedies.

Understanding Osteoporosis

Before we dive into the herbal remedy, it's crucial to understand the factors that contribute to osteoporosis. Aging, hormonal changes, nutritional deficiencies (especially calcium and vitamin D), sedentary lifestyles, and certain medical conditions can all weaken bone structure over time. Integrating herbal remedies into your health regimen can provide additional support to strengthen bones, promote mineral absorption, and enhance overall wellness.

Key Herbs for Bone Health

Several herbs have been traditionally recognized for their bone-strengthening properties. Here are a few standouts:

1. **Nettle Leaf (Urtica dioica)**: Rich in calcium, magnesium, and vitamins A and K, nettle leaf helps in mineral absorption

and may play a role in maintaining bone density.

2. **Horsetail (Equisetum arvense)**: Known for its high silica content, horsetail can help in the formation and maintenance of strong bones.
3. **Dandelion (Taraxacum officinale)**: Packed with vitamins and minerals, dandelion supports digestion and helps the body absorb nutrients more effectively.
4. **Red Clover (Trifolium pratense)**: Often used for its phytoestrogens, red clover can help address hormonal imbalances that contribute to bone loss.
5. **Turmeric (Curcuma longa)**: While primarily renowned for its anti-inflammatory properties due to curcumin, turmeric also supports bone health by aiding in calcium absorption.

An Herbal Recipe for Osteoporosis

Combining these powerful herbs can create a delicious and healthful brew that not only supports bone health but also enhances overall wellness. Here's a simple recipe you can prepare at home:

Herbal Bone Health Tea

Ingredients:

- 1 teaspoon of dried nettle leaf
- 1 teaspoon of dried horsetail
- 1 teaspoon of dried dandelion leaf
- 1 teaspoon of dried red clover flowers

- 1 teaspoon of dried turmeric root (or 1/2 teaspoon of turmeric powder)
- 4 cups of water
- Optional: Honey or lemon for flavor

Instructions:

1. **Boil Water**: In a pot, bring 4 cups of water to a gentle boil.
2. **Add Herbs**: Once the water is boiling, add the dried nettle leaf, horsetail, dandelion leaf, red clover, and turmeric. Stir gently.
3. **Simmer**: Reduce the heat to low and allow the mixture to simmer for 15-20 minutes. This step allows the active compounds in the herbs to infuse into the water.
4. **Strain**: After simmering, remove the pot from heat. Use a fine mesh strainer or a tea infuser to strain the herbs from the liquid.
5. **Add Flavor**: If desired, add honey or a squeeze of lemon for sweetness and a burst of flavor.
6. **Serve**: Pour the tea into cups and enjoy! This can be consumed warm or cooled for refreshing iced tea.

Enjoying Your Herbal Tea

Aim to drink this herbal tea 2-3 times a week to maximize its benefits for bone health. Additionally, consider incorporating other lifestyle changes, such as regular weight-bearing exercises, a balanced diet rich in calcium and vitamin D, and maintaining a healthy weight. Always consult with a healthcare provider before starting any new herbal regimen, especially if you are taking other medications or have existing health conditions.

Osteoporosis doesn't have to dictate the quality of your life. By integrating herbal remedies like the herbal bone health tea into your routine, you can nurture your bones from the inside out. Combine this tea with a balanced diet and a healthy lifestyle for optimal results. Here's to strong bones and holistic health!

61. Herbal Healing Recipe for Parkinson's Disease: Nature's Support for Wellness

Parkinson's disease (PD) is a progressive neurological disorder that primarily affects movement. While there is currently no cure, many people with Parkinson's disease seek complementary therapies to help manage symptoms and improve their quality of life. Among these, herbal remedies have gained attention for their potential benefits.

Please remember that this recipe should serve as a complementary approach and not a substitute for conventional medical treatment. Always consult your healthcare provider before starting any new herbal regimen.

Understanding Parkinson's Disease

Parkinson's disease is characterized by the loss of dopamine-producing neurons in the brain, leading to symptoms such as tremors, rigidity, and bradykinesia (slowness of movement). Additionally, individuals may experience non-motor symptoms like fatigue, depression, and cognitive changes.

Herbal remedies may aid in the management of these symptoms and promote overall well-being.

Below is a straightforward herbal recipe tailored to support your journey.

Herbal Healing Recipe: Parkinson's Serenity Tea

Ingredients:

1. **Ginger** (1 tablespoon, freshly grated)
   Ginger is known for its anti-inflammatory properties and may help alleviate nausea and movement-related discomfort.
2. **Turmeric** (1 teaspoon, ground or 1 tablespoon fresh)
   Curcumin, the active compound in turmeric, possesses potent anti-inflammatory and antioxidant properties, which can support overall brain health.
3. **Ginkgo Biloba** (1 tablespoon dried leaves)
   Ginkgo biloba is believed to improve cognitive function and circulation. It may help with memory and reduce feelings of fatigue.
4. **Lemon Balm** (1 tablespoon dried leaves)
   Known for its calming effects, lemon balm can help reduce anxiety and promote relaxation.
5. **Honey** (to taste)
   Honey not only sweetens the tea but also has antioxidant properties and supports immune health.
6. **Water** (4 cups)

Instructions:

1. **Prepare the Herbs:** If using fresh ginger and turmeric, peel and grate them. For dried herbs, measure out the necessary amounts.
2. **Boil Water:** In a pot, bring 4 cups of water to a rolling boil.
3. **Add Ingredients:** Add the grated ginger, turmeric, dried ginkgo biloba, and lemon balm to the boiling water.
4. **Simmer:** Reduce the heat and let the mixture simmer for about 10-15 minutes. This allows the herbs to infuse their beneficial properties into the water.
5. **Strain and Sweeten:** After simmering, strain the tea into a teapot or individual cups. Add honey to taste, stirring until dissolved.
6. **Serve:** Enjoy this herbal tea warm, ideally 1-2 times a day, as part of your wellness routine.

Additional Tips:

- **Maintaining a Balanced Diet:** Incorporate a variety of fruits, vegetables, whole grains, and lean proteins to support overall health.
- **Staying Active:** Regular physical activity, tailored to individual capabilities, can significantly benefit physical and mental well-being.
- **Mindfulness and Relaxation:** Practices such as yoga, tai chi, and meditation can help manage stress and anxiety, further enhancing your quality of life.

Final Thoughts

While herbal remedies can support individuals with Parkinson's disease, it's essential to approach treatment holistically. Always work with your healthcare provider to determine the best course of action tailored to your unique needs.

This herbal tea recipe offers comfort and may help with some symptoms associated with Parkinson's disease. Embrace the healing power of nature while continuing traditional medical treatments to create a balanced approach to your health. Remember, you are not alone in this journey, and support is always within reach!

Disclaimer: This herbal recipe is for informational purposes only and does not constitute medical advice. Always consult with a healthcare professional before making changes to your health regimen.

62. Herbal Healing Recipe for Alzheimer's Disease: A Natural Approach

Alzheimer's disease is a complex and challenging condition that impacts millions of individuals and families worldwide. As we search for ways to support cognitive health, herbal remedies are gaining attention for their potential benefits. While these remedies are not a cure for Alzheimer's, they may help improve memory, cognitive functions, and overall brain health.

Understanding Alzheimer's Disease

Alzheimer's disease is characterized by the progressive decline in cognitive functions, including memory, reasoning, and the ability to perform daily tasks. It is a type of dementia that affects thinking, behavior, and feelings, often leading to significant emotional distress for those diagnosed and their loved ones.

While conventional medicine focuses on managing symptoms with drugs, many people are looking to complementary approaches. These may include a combination of a healthy diet, exercise, and the use of herbs known for their neuroprotective properties.

Herbal Ingredients

Before we delve into the recipe, let's look at some beneficial herbs that have been studied for their potential effects on cognitive health:

1. **Ginkgo Biloba**: Known for enhancing blood circulation in the brain, ginkgo biloba may help improve memory and cognitive function, particularly in older adults.
2. **Bacopa Monnieri** (Brahmi): Widely used in traditional Ayurvedic medicine, Bacopa has been credited with enhancing memory and learning while reducing anxiety and stress.
3. **Turmeric**: Curcumin, the active component of turmeric, is known for its anti-inflammatory and antioxidant properties. It may help in reducing the risk of cognitive decline.
4. **Rosemary**: This fragrant herb has been linked to improved memory and concentration. Research suggests that certain compounds in rosemary may help protect against neurodegeneration.
5. **Sage**: Traditionally used for its medicinal properties, sage may help improve cognitive function and memory.

Herbal Healing Recipe

Here's a simple herbal tea blend that combines these powerful ingredients to support cognitive health. Remember, while these herbs are generally considered safe, it is essential to consult with a healthcare provider before starting any new herbal regimen, especially for individuals diagnosed with Alzheimer's disease.

Herbal Cognitive Boost Tea

Ingredients:

- 1 teaspoon dried Ginkgo Biloba leaves
- 1 teaspoon dried Bacopa Monnieri
- 1 teaspoon dried Turmeric powder (or 1-inch fresh turmeric root)
- 1 teaspoon dried Rosemary leaves
- 1 teaspoon dried Sage leaves
- 4 cups filtered water
- Honey or lemon (optional, for taste)

Instructions:

1. **Boil the Water**: In a medium saucepan, bring 4 cups of filtered water to a gentle boil.
2. **Add the Herbs**: Once boiling, reduce the heat to a simmer and add the dried Ginkgo Biloba, Bacopa, Turmeric, Rosemary, and Sage.
3. **Steep**: Allow the mixture to steep for 10-15 minutes. If using fresh turmeric, you might want to add it earlier for a richer flavor.
4. **Strain**: After steeping, strain the tea into a teapot or heatproof mug to remove the herbal particles.
5. **Serve**: Enjoy your herbal tea warm. You can enhance its flavor with a touch of honey or a squeeze of lemon if desired.

Additional Tips for a Brain-Healthy Lifestyle

Besides enjoying herbal remedies, consider incorporating these lifestyle changes to support cognitive health:

- **Balanced Diet**: Focus on a diet rich in fruits, vegetables, whole grains, healthy fats (especially omega-3 fatty acids), and lean proteins.
- **Physical Activity**: Regular exercise can enhance blood flow to the brain and improve overall health.
- **Mental Stimulation**: Engage in activities that challenge your brain, such as puzzles, reading, or learning new skills.
- **Social Interaction**: Maintain strong social connections to help reduce feelings of isolation and depression.

While the search for a cure for Alzheimer's disease continues, we can take a proactive approach to support cognitive health through natural remedies like herbal teas. The combination of Ginkgo Biloba, Bacopa Monnieri, Turmeric, Rosemary, and Sage in our Herbal Cognitive Boost Tea can serve as a gentle aid for memory support and overall brain wellness. Always consult with a healthcare professional before adding new remedies to your routine, especially for those managing Alzheimer's disease.

Be open to these natural approaches as part of a holistic lifestyle, and take small yet meaningful steps towards a healthier brain. Together, we can nurture our minds and foster hope in the face of Alzheimer's disease.

63. Herbal Healing Recipe for Nervous Shock: A Natural Approach to Recovery

Nervous shock, often characterized by feelings of anxiety, panic, and emotional distress, can occur after a traumatic event or stressful experience. In a world filled with constant pressures and unexpected challenges, many people seek natural remedies to help soothe their nerves and regain their emotional balance. Fortunately, herbal medicine offers a wealth of options that can support the body and mind during such times.

Understanding Nervous Shock

Nervous shock is a term used to describe a state of emotional disturbance that can occur after an overwhelming event. This may include accidents, the loss of a loved one, or other intense stressors. Symptoms can range from anxiety and insomnia to physical reactions like tension headaches and gastrointestinal distress.

Herbal remedies can provide gentle and effective support to help restore calm, stabilize mood, and promote overall well-being. The recipe outlined below combines herbs traditionally used for their calming and restorative properties.

The Herbal Healing Recipe

Herbal Infusion for Nervous Shock

Ingredients:

- 1 teaspoon of dried chamomile flowers
- 1 teaspoon of lemon balm leaves (Melissa officinalis)
- 1 teaspoon of passionflower (Passiflora incarnata)
- 1 teaspoon of skullcap (Scutellaria lateriflora)
- 2 cups of boiling water
- Honey (optional, for sweetness)

Instructions:

1. **Prepare the Herbs:** Gather all the dried herbs and place them in a clean, heatproof container, such as a teapot or a glass jar.
2. **Boil Water:** Bring 2 cups of fresh water to a rolling boil.
3. **Steep the Herbs:** Pour the boiling water over the herbs. Cover the container with a lid or a plate to trap the steam and essential oils. Allow the infusion to steep for 10-15 minutes.
4. **Strain the Herbs:** After steeping, strain the mixture through a fine mesh sieve or cheesecloth into a clean cup or teapot, discarding the herbs.
5. **Sweeten (Optional):** If you'd like, add a teaspoon of honey to sweeten your infusion. Honey also has soothing properties that can further support emotional calm.

6. **Enjoy the Brew:** Sip the infusion slowly, taking a moment to breathe deeply and relax as you drink.

Using the Infusion

For optimal results, consume the herbal infusion two to three times a day, especially during moments of stress or anxiety. Note that while many people benefit from herbal remedies, it is essential to listen to your body and consult with a healthcare professional if you have pre-existing conditions or are taking medication.

Learning About the Herbs

- **Chamomile:** Known for its calming effects, chamomile can help reduce anxiety and promote sleep. Its gentle nature makes it ideal for stress relief without drowsiness.
- **Lemon Balm:** This fragrant herb has both calming and uplifting properties. It can help ease feelings of sadness and anxiety while promoting relaxation.
- **Passionflower:** Often used for its sedative effects, passionflower is effective in reducing anxiety and improving sleep quality.
- **Skullcap:** A powerful herb for those experiencing nervous tension, skullcap is known to relax the nervous system and alleviate symptoms of stress.

Additional Tips for Recovery

While herbal remedies can be incredibly beneficial, it's important to approach recovery from nervous shock holistically. Here are a few additional steps you can take to support your healing journey:

- **Mindfulness and Meditation:** Practices such as mindfulness, breathing exercises, and meditation can significantly reduce anxiety and promote a sense of calm.
- **Physical Activity:** Gentle exercise like walking, yoga, or tai chi can help relieve tension in the body and boost your mood.
- **Connect with Nature:** Spend time outdoors, as nature has a rejuvenating effect on the mind and body.
- **Seek Support:** Don't hesitate to reach out to friends, family, or professionals to talk about your experience and emotions.

Herbal remedies offer a gentle yet powerful way to support your recovery from nervous shock. This herbal infusion, featuring calming ingredients like chamomile, lemon balm, passionflower, and skullcap, can help you regain your sense of peace and balance during challenging times. Remember to prioritize self-care, connect with supportive communities, and listen to your body as you navigate your healing journey. Trust the healing power of nature and take a step towards tranquility today!

64. Herbal Healing for Rheumatic Disease: A Comprehensive Recipe

Rheumatic disease encompasses a wide range of conditions that affect the joints, muscles, and connective tissues, causing pain and inflammation. Living with rheumatic disorders can be challenging, but many people find that herbal remedies can complement their treatment regimen and offer relief.

Understanding Rheumatic Disease

Before delving into the herbal remedy, it's essential to understand the nature of rheumatic diseases. Conditions such as rheumatoid arthritis, lupus, fibromyalgia, and osteoarthritis fall under this category. Individuals may experience chronic pain, stiffness, fatigue, and swelling, significantly impacting their quality of life.

While traditional medicines are often necessary for managing these conditions, many individuals are turning to natural remedies to support their health. Herbal treatments can aid in reducing inflammation, alleviating pain, and boosting overall well-being.

Herbal Remedy: Anti-Inflammatory Infusion

Ingredients

1. **Turmeric (Curcuma longa) - 1 tablespoon**
   - Known for its powerful anti-inflammatory properties due to its active compound, curcumin.
2. **Ginger (Zingiber officinale) - 1 tablespoon**
   - Contains gingerol, another potent anti-inflammatory agent, which can help to reduce pain and stiffness.
3. **Willow Bark (Salix alba) - 1 tablespoon**
   - Often referred to as "nature's aspirin," it can help relieve pain associated with inflammation.
4. **Boswellia (Boswellia serrata) - 1 tablespoon**
   - This herbal remedy is known for its ability to reduce inflammation and support joint health.
5. **Peppermint (Mentha piperita) - 1 tablespoon**
   - Provides a soothing effect and can help ease muscle tension.
6. **Honey (optional) - 1 teaspoon**
   - Acts as a natural sweetener and boasts its own anti-inflammatory properties.

Instructions

1. **Prepare the Ingredients:** Gather all the herbs and ensure they are dried and crushed if necessary. This helps release their active compounds when infused.
2. **Boil Water:** In a pot, bring about 4 cups of water to a rolling boil.

3. **Add the Herbs:** Once the water is boiling, reduce the heat to a simmer and add the turmeric, ginger, willow bark, boswellia, and peppermint.
4. **Simmer:** Let the mixture simmer for about 20 minutes. This will allow the flavors and beneficial properties of the herbs to infuse into the water.
5. **Strain:** After simmering, strain the mixture into a teapot or heat-safe container using a fine mesh strainer or cheesecloth to remove solid particles.
6. **Add Honey:** If desired, add honey to taste while the infusion is still warm. Stir well to ensure it's fully dissolved.
7. **Serve:** Pour the herbal infusion into cups and enjoy it warm.

Dosage and Usage

For best results, it is recommended to drink this herbal infusion 1-2 times a day. Regular consumption may help manage symptoms associated with rheumatic diseases. However, it is important to consult with your healthcare provider before introducing any new herbal treatments, especially if you are on prescribed medications or have underlying health conditions.

Additional Tips for Managing Rheumatic Disease

- **Stay Hydrated:** Drinking plenty of water can help support joint health and flush out toxins.

- **Dietary Considerations:** Incorporate anti-inflammatory foods like olive oil, fruits, vegetables, and fatty fish into your diet.
- **Gentle Exercise:** Activities like yoga or swimming can help maintain joint mobility without causing excessive strain.
- **Mind-Body Practices:** Consider meditation, deep breathing, or tai chi for stress reduction and pain management.

Herbal remedies can offer valuable support in managing the symptoms of rheumatic diseases. The anti-inflammatory infusion presented here combines several powerful herbs known for their health benefits. While these natural remedies can help alleviate discomfort, they should complement—not replace—traditional medical treatments. Always consult with your healthcare provider before starting any new herbal regimen, especially if you have existing medical concerns.

Remember, your journey with rheumatic disease is unique, and finding the right balance of treatment that works for you is key to achieving a better quality of life. Embrace the healing power of nature while taking charge of your health!

65. Herbal Healing Recipe for Excessive Sweating: A Natural Approach

Excessive sweating, also known as hyperhidrosis, can be an uncomfortable condition that affects various aspects of daily life. Whether it's the embarrassment of sweaty palms during a handshake, soaked clothes in a meeting, or the constant worry about odor, excessive sweating can lead to anxiety and self-consciousness. Fortunately, nature provides us with a plethora of herbs and remedies that can help manage this condition.

Below, I'll share an herbal healing recipe designed to help reduce excessive sweating. This natural remedy combines the power of herbs known for their astringent, antibacterial, and calming properties.

Understanding Excessive Sweating

Before we dive into the recipe, it's essential to understand that excessive sweating can have various triggers, including genetics, hormonal changes, and anxiety. While consulting with a healthcare professional is vital, especially if sweating is severe or sudden, herbal remedies can be a complementary approach.

Herbal Ingredients Overview

1. **Sage (Salvia officinalis)**: Known for its astringent properties, sage helps reduce sweating by constricting sweat glands. This herb is not only effective but also has antibacterial qualities that help prevent odor.
2. **Thyme (Thymus vulgaris)**: Thyme has antimicrobial properties and is believed to help with sweat regulation. Its pleasant fragrance can also provide a refreshing scent.
3. **Chamomile (Matricaria chamomilla)**: Known for its calming effects, chamomile can help ease anxiety-induced sweating. Additionally, its anti-inflammatory properties can soothe any skin irritation caused by excessive perspiration.
4. **Witch Hazel (Hamamelis virginiana)**: This natural astringent is great for treating overactive sweat glands. Often found in various skin preparations, witch hazel can help tighten pores and reduce moisture.

Herbal Healing Recipe: Sweat-Soothing Body Spray

This DIY herbal body spray is easy to make and can be applied to areas prone to excessive sweating, such as the underarms, hands, or feet. The combination of herbs not only helps control sweat production but also leaves a refreshing scent throughout the day.

Ingredients:

- **1 cup witch hazel extract**
- **1 tablespoon dried sage leaves**
- **1 tablespoon dried thyme leaves**
- **1 tablespoon dried chamomile flowers**
- **10-15 drops essential oil (optional)**: Choose oils with calming scents like lavender or tea tree oil, which also have antibacterial properties.

Instructions:

1. **Prepare an Herbal Infusion**:
   - Boil 1 cup of water and pour it over the dried sage, thyme, and chamomile in a heatproof container.
   - Cover and let it steep for about 15-20 minutes.
2. **Strain the Mixture**:
   - After steeping, use a fine mesh strainer or cheesecloth to strain the herbs from the infusion, discarding the plant materials. Allow the liquid to cool completely.
3. **Combine with Witch Hazel**:
   - Once the herbal infusion is cool, mix it with 1 cup of witch hazel in a clean spray bottle.
4. **Add Essential Oils**:
   - If desired, add 10-15 drops of your chosen essential oil to enhance the scent and benefits of the spray.
5. **Shake Well**:
   - Shake the bottle gently to combine the ingredients thoroughly.

6. **Application**:
    o Spray the mixture on areas where you experience excessive sweating, as needed. Be sure to shake the bottle before each use, as natural ingredients may settle.

Tips for Best Results

- **Patch Test**: Always do a patch test on a small area of skin to ensure no allergic reaction occurs, especially when using essential oils.
- **Daily Use**: For optimal results, use this spray daily. Consistency is key in herbal remedies.
- **Stay Hydrated**: Drinking plenty of water can also help regulate body temperature and reduce overall sweating.
- **Combine with Lifestyle Changes**: Wear breathable fabrics, avoid spicy foods, and manage stress through practices like yoga or meditation for added support against excessive sweating.

Final Thought

While excessive sweating can be challenging to deal with, herbal remedies offer a natural and holistic approach to management. This sweat-soothing body spray encapsulates the healing power of nature and can help you feel more confident and comfortable in your skin. Recognize the power of plants, and let nature guide you on your path to balance!

66. Herbal Healing for Arterial Compression: A Natural Recipe for Relief

In our fast-paced world, heart health is more critical than ever. Many individuals face various cardiovascular issues, including arterial compression, which can lead to discomfort and reduced blood flow. While clinical treatments are always important, many people seek natural remedies to complement their healthcare regimen. Today, we will explore an herbal healing recipe aimed at providing relief from arterial compression.

Understanding Arterial Compression

Arterial compression occurs when arteries become narrowed or constrained, often leading to restricted blood flow. This condition can result from various factors, including inflammation, buildup of plaque, or external pressure on the vessels from surrounding tissues. Symptoms can vary but often include pain, cramping, fatigue, and numbness in the affected areas.

While it's essential to consult a healthcare professional for a proper diagnosis and treatment plan, integrating herbal remedies into your life can support vascular health and alleviate discomfort.

Herbal Ingredients for Arterial Compression

Before we dive into our healing recipe, let's see some key herbs known for their beneficial effects on circulatory health:

1. Ginger (Zingiber officinale)

Ginger is renowned for its ability to enhance circulation and reduce inflammation. This warming herb can help relax blood vessels and improve blood flow, making it an excellent addition to any herbal remedy aimed at supporting arterial health.

2. Turmeric (Curcuma longa)

Turmeric contains curcumin, a powerful compound with antioxidant and anti-inflammatory properties. Curcumin can help improve endothelial function and reduce arterial stiffness, making turmeric a valuable herb for promoting cardiovascular health.

3. Garlic (Allium sativum)

Garlic has long been celebrated for its heart health benefits. It can help lower blood pressure, reduce cholesterol levels, and improve circulation.

4. Cayenne Pepper (Capsicum annuum)

Cayenne is known for its ability to stimulate circulation and enhance the flow of blood throughout the body. It contains capsaicin, which can help improve arterial function.

5. Hawthorn (Crataegus spp.)

Hawthorn berries and leaves have been used for centuries to support heart health. They improve blood flow, reduce blood pressure, and enhance the overall functioning of the cardiovascular system.

A Healing Herbal Infusion for Arterial Compression

Ingredients:

- 1 teaspoon dried ginger root or 1-inch piece of fresh ginger (sliced)
- 1 teaspoon dried turmeric root or 1-inch piece of fresh turmeric (sliced)
- 2 cloves of garlic (minced)
- 1/2 teaspoon cayenne pepper
- 1 tablespoon hawthorn berries (dried)
- 4 cups of water
- Honey (optional, to taste)
- Lemon juice (optional, for flavor)

Instructions:

1. **Prepare Your Ingredients**: Gather all the herbs and spices. If you're using fresh ginger or turmeric, peel and slice them accordingly.
2. **Boil Water**: In a medium-sized pot, bring the 4 cups of water to a boil.

3. **Add Ingredients**: Once the water is boiling, add the ginger, turmeric, garlic, cayenne pepper, and hawthorn berries to the pot.
4. **Simmer**: Reduce the heat and let the mixture simmer for about 20 minutes. This allows the active compounds of the herbs to infuse the water.
5. **Strain the Mixture**: After simmering, strain the infusion into a teapot or a heatproof container to remove the solid herbs.
6. **Optional Additions**: If desired, sweeten with honey and add a splash of lemon juice for flavor.
7. **Serve**: Enjoy this herbal infusion warm. For best results, drink 1-2 cups a day.

While herbal remedies can provide supportive care for arterial compression, it's important to remember that they should not replace medical treatment or professional advice. This herbal infusion, rich in anti-inflammatory and circulation-supporting properties, can be a lovely addition to your health routine. Embrace the power of nature, and take steps toward heart health the herbal way!

Remember:

A balanced diet, regular physical activity, and a healthy lifestyle are the best ways to promote overall cardiovascular health.

67. Herbal Healing for Restless Leg Syndrome: A Natural Recipe to Find Relief

Restless Leg Syndrome (RLS) is a condition that affects millions of people around the world, characterized by an uncontrollable urge to move the legs, often accompanied by uncomfortable sensations. This can lead to sleepless nights and a significant impact on quality of life. While conventional medicine offers various treatments, many individuals seek natural remedies to alleviate their symptoms.

Understanding Restless Leg Syndrome

Before diving into our herbal remedy, let's take a moment to understand RLS. Symptoms can vary from mild to severe and typically worsen during periods of inactivity, particularly in the evening or while trying to sleep. People with RLS often describe sensations like tingling, crawling, or burning in their legs, and movement usually brings temporary relief.

Natural Ingredients for RLS Relief

Several herbs and natural ingredients have shown promise in relieving RLS symptoms. The following herbs mentioned in our recipe are known for their soothing and calming properties:

1. **Valerian Root**: Renowned for its calming effects, valerian can help improve sleep quality and reduce anxiety, which can exacerbate RLS symptoms.
2. **Passionflower**: This herb is known for its mild sedative effects and can help reduce restlessness and promote relaxation.
3. **Magnesium**: While not an herb, magnesium deficiency is often linked to muscle cramps and spasms. Supplementing with magnesium or using it topically can help alleviate symptoms.
4. **Ginger**: Known for its anti-inflammatory properties, ginger can assist in reducing discomfort in the legs and help with overall circulation.
5. **Chamomile**: With its calming effects, chamomile tea can promote relaxation before sleep and soothe nervous tension.

Herbal Healing Recipe for RLS

Here's a soothing herbal tea recipe that combines these beneficial ingredients to provide relief from Restless Leg Syndrome:

Restful Leg Herbal Tea
Ingredients:

- 1 teaspoon dried valerian root
- 1 teaspoon dried passionflower
- 1 teaspoon dried chamomile flowers
- 1 teaspoon grated fresh ginger (or 1/2 teaspoon dried ginger)
- 1 cup water

- Honey or lemon (optional, for taste)
- A pinch of magnesium (such as magnesium citrate powder; consult with a healthcare professional for proper dosage)

Instructions:

1. **Boil Water**: In a small pot, bring 1 cup of water to a boil.
2. **Add Herbs**: Once boiling, remove the pot from the heat and add the valerian root, passionflower, chamomile, and ginger.
3. **Steep**: Cover the pot with a lid and allow the herbs to steep for 10-15 minutes.
4. **Strain**: After steeping, strain the tea into a cup. If desired, add honey or lemon to enhance the flavor.
5. **Incorporate Magnesium**: If using magnesium, stir in a pinch into the tea. Ensure you are following appropriate guidelines for dosage, and consult a healthcare provider as needed.
6. **Enjoy**: Sip your herbal tea in the evening, ideally about 30-60 minutes before bedtime, to help relax and prepare for restful sleep.

Additional Tips for Managing RLS

While herbal remedies can be effective in managing RLS symptoms, there are other lifestyle changes and practices to consider:

- **Regular Exercise**: Engage in regular physical activity during the day to help decrease RLS symptoms.
- **Avoid Caffeine and Alcohol**: These substances can increase RLS symptoms, particularly when consumed later in the day.
- **Establish a Sleep Routine**: Create a calming pre-sleep ritual to help signal your body that it's time to rest.

Finding relief from Restless Leg Syndrome can be a journey, and while herbal remedies may not replace conventional treatments, they can be a wonderful complementary approach. By integrating this soothing herbal tea into your nightly routine, you can promote relaxation and potentially ease the discomfort associated with RLS. Always consult with a healthcare professional before making significant changes to your health regimen, and enjoy the journey towards restful nights and peaceful legs!

68. Herbal Healing for Urinary Tract Infections (UTIs): A Natural Recipe

Urinary tract infections (UTIs) are among the most common health issues that affect millions of people every year. While traditional treatments often involve antibiotics, many are turning to herbal remedies for a more natural approach. Herbal medicine has been used for centuries to support urinary health, and several herbs can target the symptoms and causes of UTIs effectively.

Understanding UTIs

Before diving into the recipe, it's essential to understand what a UTI is and what contributes to its occurrence. UTIs can affect any part of the urinary system: the bladder, kidneys, ureters, or urethra. Symptoms typically include:

- A strong, persistent urge to urinate
- A burning sensation during urination
- Frequent urination
- Cloudy or strong-smelling urine
- Pelvic pain in women
- Rectal pain in men

Several factors contribute to UTIs, such as dehydration, poor hygiene, and certain lifestyle choices. Always consult a healthcare professional if you suspect you have a UTI, as untreated infections can lead to more severe health issues.

The Power of Herbs

Herbs have unique properties that can help prevent and treat UTIs. Some of the most effective herbs for urinary health include:

- **Cranberry:** Known for its ability to prevent bacteria from adhering to the bladder wall.
- **Dandelion:** Acts as a diuretic and promotes kidney function.
- **Uva Ursi (Bearberry):** Contains compounds that can inhibit the growth of bacteria in the urinary tract.
- **Nettle:** Supports kidney function and promotes urination.
- **Peppermint:** Soothes irritation and is an antispasmodic.

Herbal Healing Recipe: UTI Tincture

This herbal tincture combines the healing properties of several potent herbs to create a powerful natural remedy for UTIs.

Ingredients:

- 1 part dried cranberry (Vaccinium macrocarpon)
- 1 part dried uva ursi (Arctostaphylos uva-ursi)
- 1 part dried nettle leaf (Urtica dioica)

- 1 part dried dandelion root (Taraxacum officinale)
- 1 part dried peppermint leaf (Mentha piperita)
- 80 proof vodka or food-grade vegetable glycerin (for a glycerin-based tincture)
- A mason jar with a tight-fitting lid

Instructions:

1. **Prepare Your Ingredients:** Ensure all dried herbs are of good quality and free from contaminants. You can purchase these at health food stores or herbal shops.
2. **Combine the Herbs:** In your mason jar, add equal parts of dried cranberry, uva ursi, nettle, dandelion root, and peppermint leaf. The ratios can be adjusted based on preference, but using equal parts helps balance their properties.
3. **Add the Base:** Pour the vodka or glycerin over the herbs until they are fully submerged. Leave about an inch of space at the top of the jar.
4. **Seal and Shake:** Seal the jar tightly and shake it well to mix the contents. Store the jar in a cool, dark place, shaking it daily for at least 4-6 weeks. This process allows the herbal constituents to infuse into the liquid.
5. **Strain and Bottle:** After the infusion period, strain the mixture using a fine mesh strainer or cheesecloth. Discard the herbs and transfer the liquid to a dropper bottle for easy use.

How to Use:

Take **10-15 drops** of the tincture in a small glass of water **up to three times per day** during an active UTI or as a preventative measure. Make sure to consult with a healthcare professional before starting any new herbal regimen, especially if you are pregnant, nursing, or taking other medications.

Additional Tips for UTI Prevention

In addition to using herbal remedies, incorporating lifestyle changes can help prevent UTIs:

- **Hydration:** Drink plenty of water to dilute urine and flush out bacteria.
- **Hygiene:** Wipe from front to back after using the bathroom and urinate after sexual intercourse.
- **Cranberry Juice:** Unsweetened cranberry juice can help prevent the buildup of bacteria in the urinary tract.
- **Cotton Underwear:** Wearing breathable underwear may promote better moisture control.

Herbal healing offers a gentle yet effective approach to managing and preventing UTIs. This herbal tincture recipe can serve as a valuable tool in your natural wellness toolkit, but remember that it is essential to consult with a healthcare provider for serious symptoms or recurring infections. By combining herbal remedies with healthy lifestyle choices, you can support your urinary health naturally and effectively.

Cheers to your health!

69. Herbal Healing for Gastroenteritis: A Soothing Recipe

Gastroenteritis, commonly known as stomach flu, is often caused by infections from bacteria, viruses, or parasites. Symptoms typically include diarrhea, vomiting, abdominal cramps, and fatigue. While conventional medicine plays an essential role in managing these symptoms, many people turn to herbal remedies for support. Below, we will explore an herbal healing recipe that can help alleviate discomfort and promote recovery from gastroenteritis.

What Is Gastroenteritis?

Before delving into herbal remedies, let's briefly understand gastroenteritis. It is an inflammation of the stomach and intestines, often resulting in the rapid onset of symptoms. Infection can occur through contaminated food or water, or close contact with infected individuals. Staying hydrated and resting are crucial aspects of recovery, but adding herbal remedies may offer additional relief.

Herbal Ingredients with Healing Properties

1. Ginger

Ginger is renowned for its digestive benefits, particularly in alleviating nausea and vomiting.

Its anti-inflammatory properties can help soothe the gastrointestinal tract and promote comfort.

2. Chamomile

Chamomile is known for its calming effects and can aid in reducing bloating and cramping. It also has mild antibacterial properties, making it beneficial in combating stomach infections.

3. Peppermint

Peppermint is another excellent herb for digestive health. It helps relax the muscles of the gastrointestinal tract, reducing cramping and discomfort. Additionally, peppermint tea can provide a refreshing taste while soothing nausea.

4. Licorice Root

Licorice root has been traditionally used to support digestive health. Its anti-inflammatory and soothing properties may help protect the stomach lining and promote overall healing.

5. Fennel Seeds

Fennel seeds are known for their carminative properties, which help relieve gas, bloating, and discomfort. They also have antimicrobial properties that can aid in combating infections.

A Soothing Herbal Tea Recipe for Gastroenteritis

Ingredients:

- 1 teaspoon dried ginger (or ½ teaspoon fresh ginger, grated)
- 1 teaspoon dried chamomile flowers
- 1 teaspoon dried peppermint leaves
- 1 teaspoon fennel seeds
- ½ teaspoon dried licorice root (optional)
- 4 cups of water
- Honey (optional, for taste)

Instructions:

1. **Boil the Water**: In a medium pot, bring 4 cups of water to a rolling boil.
2. **Add Herbs**: Once boiling, turn off the heat and add the ginger, chamomile, peppermint, fennel seeds, and licorice root (if using). Stir to combine.
3. **Steep**: Cover the pot and let the mixture steep for about 10-15 minutes. This allows the herbs to release their beneficial properties into the water.
4. **Strain and Serve**: Using a fine mesh strainer, strain the tea into a teapot or directly into cups. Add honey if desired for sweetness.
5. **Enjoy**: Sip the tea slowly while it's still warm. This tea can be consumed 2-3 times a day, especially when experiencing symptoms.

Additional Tips:

- **Stay Hydrated**: It's important to drink plenty of fluids. In addition to herbal tea, consider clear broths or electrolyte solutions to replenish lost fluids.
- **Diet Consideration**: As your stomach begins to settle, introduce bland foods such as toast, rice, or bananas to help ease your digestive system back to normal.

When to Seek Medical Attention

While herbal remedies can be supportive during recovery, it's essential to recognize when to seek medical assistance. If symptoms persist beyond a few days, or if you experience severe dehydration, high fever, or blood in your stool, consult a healthcare professional promptly.

Herbal remedies can be a gentle and effective way to support your body during an episode of gastroenteritis. The soothing tea recipe provided can help ease discomfort, reduce nausea, and promote relaxation. Remember to prioritize hydration and rest for optimal recovery.

70. Herbal Healing for High Cholesterol: A Natural Recipe to Lower Your Levels

In today's fast-paced world, maintaining heart health is more important than ever. High cholesterol is a prevalent condition that can lead to serious complications like heart disease and stroke. While conventional medicine offers various pharmaceutical solutions, many people are turning to herbal remedies for a more natural approach.

Understanding High Cholesterol

Cholesterol is a waxy substance produced by the liver that's essential for various bodily functions, including hormone production and cell membrane integrity. However, when cholesterol levels become too high—especially low-density lipoprotein (LDL) cholesterol, often referred to as "bad" cholesterol—this can lead to plaque buildup in the arteries, increasing the risk of cardiovascular disease.

Maintaining a balance of cholesterol levels through diet, exercise, and lifestyle choices is crucial. Alongside traditional treatments, certain herbs are known for their cholesterol-lowering properties, making them a valuable addition to your overall management strategy.

An Herbal Healing Recipe: The Cholesterol-Reducing Tea

This herbal tea is packed with ingredients known for their beneficial effects on cholesterol levels. It combines the power of garlic, ginger, turmeric, and green tea—a potent blend that not only supports heart health but also enhances your overall well-being.

Ingredients

- **1 clove of garlic** (crushed)
- **1 inch of fresh ginger root** (grated)
- **1 teaspoon of turmeric powder** (or fresh turmeric, grated)
- **1 green tea bag** (or 1 teaspoon of loose-leaf green tea)
- **2 cups of water**
- **Honey** (optional, for sweetness)
- **Lemon juice** (optional, for added flavor and vitamin C)

Instructions

1. **Prepare the Ingredients**: Start by crushing the garlic and grating the ginger and turmeric. These fresh ingredients release powerful compounds when crushed or grated.
2. **Boil the Water**: In a saucepan, bring 2 cups of water to a boil.
3. **Add the Ingredients**: Once the water is boiling, add the crushed garlic, grated ginger, and turmeric powder to the pan.

Reduce the heat and let the mixture simmer for about 10 minutes.

4. **Steep the Green Tea**: After simmering, remove the pan from heat and add the green tea bag (or loose-leaf tea in a strainer) to the mixture. Allow it to steep for 3-5 minutes.
5. **Strain and Serve**: Strain the tea into a mug. If desired, add a teaspoon of honey for sweetness and a splash of lemon juice for flavor.
6. **Enjoy**: Sip your herbal tea once a day. It can be enjoyed warm or chilled, depending on your preference.

Benefits of the Key Ingredients

- **Garlic**: Contains allicin, which has been shown to lower total cholesterol and LDL cholesterol levels. Garlic also has antioxidant and anti-inflammatory properties.
- **Ginger**: Known to improve circulation and help reduce cholesterol levels, ginger also aids in digestion and has anti-inflammatory benefits.
- **Turmeric**: Curcumin, the active compound in turmeric, can help reduce cholesterol levels and has potent anti-inflammatory properties, supporting overall heart health.
- **Green Tea**: Rich in catechins and antioxidants, green tea has been linked to lower cholesterol levels and overall improved cardiovascular health.

Additional Lifestyle Tips for Managing Cholesterol

1. **Diet**: Incorporate more fruits, vegetables, whole grains, and healthy fats (like olive oil and avocado) while reducing saturated and trans fats.
2. **Exercise**: Aim for at least 150 minutes of moderate aerobic activity each week, such as brisk walking or cycling.
3. **Manage Stress**: Practice relaxation techniques like yoga or meditation to help manage stress, which can affect cholesterol levels.
4. **Quit Smoking**: If you smoke, quitting can improve your HDL ("good" cholesterol) levels and benefit your overall heart health.
5. **Regular Check-ups**: Keep track of your cholesterol levels through regular health check-ups and consultations with healthcare professionals.

Herbal remedies can play a significant role in managing high cholesterol levels naturally. This herbal healing recipe is an excellent addition to your daily routine but should not replace professional medical advice. Always consult your healthcare provider before making any major changes to your diet or starting new herbal remedies, especially if you are on medication.

By combining this herbal tea with a healthy lifestyle, you can take proactive steps toward better heart health and well-being. So brew a cup today and embrace the journey to a healthier you!

71. Herbal Healing Recipe for Meningitis: A Natural Approach to Support Recovery

Meningitis, an inflammation of the protective membranes covering the brain and spinal cord, can be a serious condition requiring immediate medical attention. While it is crucial to seek professional medical help if you or someone you know is experiencing symptoms of meningitis, some herbal remedies can provide supportive care alongside traditional treatments.

Understanding Meningitis

Meningitis can be caused by viral, bacterial, or fungal infections. Symptoms can include sudden fever, headache, stiff neck, sensitivity to light, confusion, and sometimes a rash. If you suspect meningitis, it's essential to get medical help immediately. Herbal remedies should never replace conventional treatment but can be used to complement it under professional guidance.

Herbal Healing Recipe: Soothing Meningitis Support Tea

Ingredients

1. **Echinacea** (Echinacea purpurea) – 2 teaspoons (dried or fresh)

- o Known for its immune-boosting properties, echinacea can help in fighting off infections.
2. **Ginger root** (Zingiber officinale) – 1 teaspoon (freshly grated)
   - o Ginger is anti-inflammatory and can ease headaches and nausea that may accompany meningitis.
3. **Peppermint leaves** (Mentha piperita) – 1 teaspoon (dried)
   - o Peppermint can provide relief from headaches and can also help soothe digestive issues.
4. **Lemon balm** (Melissa officinalis) – 1 teaspoon (dried)
   - o This herb helps in reducing anxiety and promoting relaxation, which can be beneficial during recovery.
5. **Honey** – 1 to 2 tablespoons (to taste)
   - o Honey has soothing properties and provides natural sweetness, enhancing flavor and providing energy.
6. **Filtered water** – 2 cups

Instructions

1. **Prepare the Ingredients:**
   - o If using fresh ginger, peel and grate it. Measure out the dried herbs and have them ready.
2. **Boil the Water:**
   - o In a small pot, bring 2 cups of filtered water to boil.
3. **Add the Herbs:**

- o Once the water has reached a boil, reduce the heat and add the echinacea, ginger, peppermint, and lemon balm.
4. **Steep the Tea:**
   - o Allow the mix to steep for about 10-15 minutes. The longer it steeps, the more potent the tea will be.
5. **Strain and Serve:**
   - o After steeping, strain the tea into a cup. Add honey to taste, stirring until dissolved.
6. **Enjoy Warm:**
   - o This soothing tea can be enjoyed warm, and you can drink it 2-3 times daily.

Notes on Usage

- **Consult Your Healthcare Provider:** Always consult with a healthcare provider before starting any herbal remedy, especially in the case of serious conditions like meningitis.
- **Stay Hydrated:** Herbal teas can be hydrating, but maintaining adequate fluid intake with water and other clear fluids is crucial.
- **Combination with Treatment:** Use this tea as a supportive remedy alongside prescribed medications but do not use it as a substitute.

Additional Supportive Practices

Besides the herbal tea, consider incorporating the following supportive practices into your routine:

- **Rest and Relaxation:** Getting plenty of rest is essential for recovery. Create a calm environment that promotes relaxation.
- **Nutritious Diet:** Focus on a balanced diet rich in antioxidants, vitamins, and minerals. Foods like fruits, vegetables, nuts, and seeds can help strengthen the immune system.
- **Gentle Movement:** If energy levels allow, gentle stretching or yoga can help alleviate tension in the body.
- **Mindfulness and Stress Reduction:** Techniques such as deep breathing, meditation, or gentle mindfulness can help manage stress levels.

While an herbal remedy like the soothing Meningitis Support Tea can assist in promoting comfort and wellness, it is vital to remember that the approval and guidance of healthcare professionals are paramount when dealing with this serious condition. Always place your health and safety first, and complement any treatment case with supportive natural practices where appropriate.

72. Embracing Nature's Remedies: An Herbal Healing Recipe for Arthritis

Arthritis, a condition affecting millions around the globe, is characterized by inflammation, pain, and stiffness in the joints. While conventional medicine offers a range of treatments, many individuals seek natural alternatives to ease their symptoms. Mother Nature has an arsenal of herbs that can provide relief and support joint health.

Understanding the Power of Herbs

Herbs have been used for centuries in traditional medicine for their potential to heal and soothe various ailments. For arthritis, specific herbs are known for their anti-inflammatory, analgesic (pain-relieving), and antioxidant properties. Some of the most effective herbs for arthritis include:

- **Turmeric**: Contains curcumin, which has potent anti-inflammatory properties.
- **Ginger**: Known for its ability to reduce inflammation and alleviate pain.
- **Willow Bark**: Contains salicin, a compound similar to aspirin, which helps with pain relief.
- **Boswellia**: A powerful anti-inflammatory herb commonly used in Ayurvedic medicine.

- **Devil's Claw**: Known for its ability to relieve pain and inflammation.

Herbal Healing Recipe for Arthritis

Anti-Inflammatory Herbal Tea

This simple, soothing herbal tea combines many of the aforementioned ingredients to create a powerful anti-inflammatory remedy.

Ingredients:

- 1 teaspoon dried turmeric root (or 1/2 teaspoon turmeric powder)
- 1 teaspoon dried ginger root (or 1/2 teaspoon ginger powder)
- 1 teaspoon dried willow bark
- 1 teaspoon dried boswellia
- 1 teaspoon dried devil's claw
- 2 cups water
- Honey or lemon (optional for taste)

Instructions:

1. **Prepare the Herbs**: If you're using whole dried roots, chop them into smaller pieces to help release their medicinal properties.
2. **Boil the Water**: In a saucepan, bring 2 cups of water to a boil.
3. **Combine and Simmer**: Once the water has reached a rolling boil, add in the turmeric, ginger, willow bark, boswellia, and devil's claw. Reduce the heat and let the mixture simmer for about 15–20 minutes.

4. **Strain the Tea**: After simmering, remove
   the saucepan from the heat. Strain the tea
   into a cup using a fine mesh strainer or
   cheesecloth to remove the herbs.
5. **Add Flavor (Optional)**: If desired, sweeten
   your tea with honey or add a squeeze of
   lemon for a refreshing twist.
6. **Enjoy**: Sip on this herbal tea once or twice
   a day to help manage arthritis symptoms
   and support joint health.

Important Tips:

- **Consult with a Healthcare Provider**:
  Always consult your healthcare provider
  before trying new herbal remedies,
  especially if you are on medication or have
  existing health concerns.
- **Stay Consistent**: Herbal treatments may
  take time to show effects. Consistency is
  key.
- **Diet and Lifestyle**: Consider incorporating
  a balanced diet rich in anti-inflammatory
  foods (like fruits, vegetables, nuts, and
  whole grains) and engage in regular, low-
  impact exercise to further support joint
  health.

Living with arthritis can be a challenge, but with
the right approach and natural remedies, it's
possible to manage and alleviate symptoms. This
herbal tea recipe is a delightful way to harness
the therapeutic benefits of nature's bounty to
support your joints. Embrace the healing power of

herbs and take a step towards a more comfortable life with arthritis.

73. An Herbal Healing Recipe for Whooping Cough: Nature's Remedy

Whooping cough, known scientifically as pertussis, is a highly contagious respiratory disease characterized by severe coughing fits. While modern medicine offers various treatments and vaccines, many people are turning to herbal remedies for relief.

Understanding Whooping Cough

Before diving into herbal remedies, it's important to understand whooping cough better. Caused by the bacterium *Bordetella pertussis*, whooping cough is particularly dangerous for infants and can lead to complications like pneumonia. Symptoms typically begin with a mild cold that develops into intense coughing fits, often producing a "whooping" sound as the patient inhales.

If you or someone you know is suffering from whooping cough, it is paramount to consult a healthcare professional for a proper diagnosis and treatment plan. However, complementary herbal remedies can be used to ease discomfort and support the healing process.

An Herbal Healing Recipe: Soothing Cough Syrup

The following herbal syrup recipe combines ingredients known for their cough-relieving and soothing properties. Please note that this herbal remedy can be used to help relieve symptoms but should not replace medical treatment.

Ingredients:

- 1 cup water
- 1 tablespoon dried marshmallow root (Althaea officinalis)
- 1 tablespoon dried thyme (Thymus vulgaris)
- 1 tablespoon dried licorice root (Glycyrrhiza glabra) – use caution if you have hypertension
- 1 tablespoon honey (optional for children over one year of age)
- Juice of half a lemon

Instructions:

1. **Prepare the Herbal Infusion:**
   - In a small pot, bring 1 cup of water to a gentle boil.
   - Once boiling, add the dried marshmallow root, thyme, and licorice root.
   - Reduce the heat and let it simmer for about 15-20 minutes. This allows the medicinal properties of the herbs to be extracted into the water.
2. **Strain the Mixture:**
   - After simmering, remove the pot from the heat and strain the liquid into a glass jar or bowl, discarding the solid

herbs. You should have a fragrant herbal infusion.

3. **Add Honey and Lemon:**
   - While the infusion is still warm (but not boiling), stir in the honey and lemon juice. Honey acts as a natural sweetener and has antimicrobial properties, while lemon provides vitamin C and helps to thin mucus.
4. **Cool and Store:**
   - Allow the syrup to cool completely before transferring it to a clean glass jar with a lid. Store it in the refrigerator for up to two weeks.

How to Use the Herbal Syrup

- **Dosage for Adults:** One tablespoon several times daily as needed.
- **Dosage for Children:** Half a teaspoon to one teaspoon no more than three times a day (consult a pediatrician for infants or young children).

Additional Herbal Remedies

While the above syrup is effective, other herbs can complement your treatment for whooping cough:

- **Peppermint:** Known for its soothing and cooling properties, peppermint tea can help relax the throat and reduce coughing fits.
- **Throat Coat Tea:** Formulations containing slippery elm and licorice may help coat the throat and reduce irritation.

- **Ginger:** Fresh ginger tea can alleviate soreness and has anti-inflammatory properties.

Important Precautions

- Always check with a healthcare professional before starting any herbal remedies, especially if you are pregnant, nursing, have existing health conditions, or are on medication.
- Ensure that honey is not given to children under one year of age due to the risk of botulism.
- Monitor symptoms closely and seek medical attention if they worsen.

Herbal remedies can provide comfort and potentially aid in the recovery from whooping cough by alleviating symptoms and supporting the body's immune response. The soothing cough syrup we've discussed is an easy and natural way to help manage coughing fits and throat irritation. Remember to use this herbal remedy as a complementary approach and prioritize medical advice and treatment for the best outcomes.

Stay healthy, and may the healing powers of nature support you on your journey to recovery!

74. Herbal Healing Recipe for Food Poisoning: Natural Remedies to Soothe Your Stomach

Food poisoning can be a serious and uncomfortable experience, often caused by consuming contaminated food or beverages. Symptoms like nausea, vomiting, diarrhea, and abdominal pain can leave you feeling drained and helpless. While it's crucial to consult a healthcare professional if symptoms persist or worsen, there are several herbal remedies that can help soothe mild cases of food poisoning. Below, I'll share an herbal healing recipe that can aid in recovery and restore your digestive health.

Understanding Food Poisoning

Food poisoning is a result of ingesting harmful bacteria, viruses, or parasites. Common culprits include undercooked meats, contaminated produce, and improperly stored foods. Symptoms can appear within hours or days of consumption, and while most cases resolve on their own, the discomfort can be significant.

Herbal Healing: The Power of Nature

Herbs have been used for centuries in various cultures around the world for their healing properties. Many herbs have anti-inflammatory, antibacterial, and soothing attributes that can alleviate symptoms associated with food poisoning. The following recipe combines several potent herbs known for their healing benefits.

Herbal Healing Recipe: Soothing Ginger-Mint Tea

This fragrant tea harnesses the soothing properties of ginger and mint, both known to ease digestive distress. Ginger is excellent for reducing nausea and inflammation, while peppermint can aid in calming the stomach muscles and relieving gastrointestinal discomfort.

Ingredients

- **1 tablespoon fresh ginger** (peeled and sliced or grated)
- **1 tablespoon fresh mint leaves** (or 1 teaspoon dried peppermint)
- **2 cups water**
- **1 tablespoon honey** (optional, for soothing sweetness)
- **Fresh lemon juice** (optional, for added flavor and vitamin C)

Instructions

1. **Boil the Water**: In a small saucepan, bring 2 cups of water to a boil.
2. **Add the Ingredients**: Once boiling, add the sliced ginger and mint leaves. If using dried

peppermint, simply add it to the boiling
water.

3. **Simmer**: Reduce the heat and let the
   mixture simmer for about 10–15 minutes.
   This allows the flavors and healing
   properties to infuse into the water.
4. **Strain**: After simmering, strain the tea into
   a cup to remove the solid pieces of ginger
   and mint.
5. **Add Sweetener and Lemon**: If desired, stir
   in honey and a squeeze of fresh lemon juice
   to taste.
6. **Enjoy**: Sip the tea slowly, allowing the
   warmth to soothe your stomach.

Additional Herbal Support

While ginger and mint are powerful allies, there
are other herbs you can consider incorporating
into your recovery regimen:

- **Chamomile**: Known for its calming effects,
  chamomile can help relax the digestive tract
  and ease stomach cramps.
- **Fennel Seeds**: Chewing on fennel seeds or
  making fennel tea can help relieve bloating
  and gas, further aiding digestion.
- **Turmeric**: This anti-inflammatory spice can
  be added to warm water or smoothies for an
  additional boost.

Tips for Recovery

- **Stay Hydrated**: It's essential to drink
  plenty of fluids, especially if you're

experiencing vomiting or diarrhea. Herbal teas, clear broths, and electrolyte solutions can help keep you hydrated.
- **Listen to Your Body**: Eat bland foods that are easy to digest, such as toast, rice, applesauce, and bananas, once you feel up to eating.
- **Rest**: Recovery takes time, so give your body the opportunity to heal.

When to Seek Medical Help

While herbal remedies can be beneficial, it's important to know when to seek medical assistance. If symptoms persist for more than 48 hours, are severe, or are accompanied by high fever, blood in vomit or stool, or signs of dehydration (such as excessive thirst, dry mouth, or dizziness), please consult a healthcare professional immediately.

Food poisoning can be a real downer, but with the right herbal remedies and self-care practices, you can support your body's healing process. The soothing ginger-mint tea recipe is a gentle yet effective way to alleviate symptoms and promote relaxation. Remember, nature has provided us with powerful tools to aid in our recovery, and with a little patience and care, you'll be back on your feet in no time.

Stay healthy and take care of your digestive wellness!

75. Herbal Healing: A Recipe for Heart Health after a Heart Attack

Heart disease remains one of the leading causes of mortality worldwide, making heart health a crucial aspect of overall well-being. While conventional medicine plays a vital role in treating heart issues, many individuals turn to natural remedies to complement their healing journey. This information presents an herbal healing recipe designed to support recovery after a heart attack. Please note that this recipe should be used in conjunction with professional medical advice.

Understanding Heart Health

Before diving into herbal remedies, it's essential to acknowledge the significance of a healthy lifestyle in preventing heart disease. A balanced diet, regular exercise, stress management, and avoiding tobacco and excessive alcohol consumption are vital components of heart health. Herbs can serve as valuable allies in this journey.

A Heart-Friendly Herbal Blend

This herbal remedy focuses on ingredients known for their cardiovascular benefits. It aims to promote heart health, improve circulation, and reduce inflammation while nourishing the body. The following recipe can be incorporated into your daily routine, but always discuss any new herbal treatments with your healthcare provider, especially after a heart attack.

Ingredients:
1. **Hawthorn Berries** (Crataegus spp.) – 1 tablespoon
   - Known for improving blood circulation and reducing blood pressure. Hawthorn also strengthens the heart muscle.
2. **Ginger Root** (Zingiber officinale) – 1 teaspoon, fresh or dried
   - Acts as an anti-inflammatory and may help lower cholesterol levels. Ginger also supports digestion and circulation.
3. **Turmeric** (Curcuma longa) – 1 teaspoon, ground
   - This powerful anti-inflammatory herb contains curcumin, which has been linked to various heart health benefits, including improved endothelial function.
4. **Garlic** (Allium sativum) – 1 clove, minced or 1 teaspoon, dried powder
   - Garlic may help lower blood pressure and reduce cholesterol levels, both of which are essential for heart health.
5. **Cinnamon** (Cinnamomum verum) – ½ teaspoon, ground
   - Beneficial for regulating blood sugar levels and has anti-inflammatory properties.
6. **Lemon** – Juice of ½ lemon

- o Fresh lemon juice adds vitamin C, supports digestion, and may help lower blood pressure.
7. **Raw Honey** – 1 teaspoon (optional)
   - o A natural sweetener that may enhance immunity and provide energy.
8. **Water – 4 cups**

Instructions:

1. **Prepare the Herbal Infusion:**
   - o In a saucepan, bring 4 cups of water to a boil. Add the hawthorn berries, ginger root, turmeric, garlic, and cinnamon to the boiling water. Reduce the heat and let the mixture simmer for about 15-20 minutes.
2. **Strain and Sweeten:**
   - o After simmering, remove the saucepan from the heat. Use a fine mesh strainer or cheesecloth to strain the liquid into a heatproof container. If desired, add raw honey for sweetness and mix well.
3. **Add Lemon Juice:**
   - o Allow the infusion to cool for a few minutes, then stir in the fresh lemon juice.
4. **Store and Serve:**
   - o You can drink the infusion warm or allow it to cool completely and store it in the refrigerator for up to three days. Enjoy a cup daily as part of your heart-healthy routine.

Additional Tips for Heart Health

While this herbal infusion can be beneficial, remember that a wholesome lifestyle is essential for heart recovery. Here are some additional tips:

- **Diet**: Emphasize whole foods, including fruits, vegetables, whole grains, lean proteins, and healthy fats. Omega-3 fatty acids found in fish, flaxseeds, and walnuts can also support heart health.
- **Hydration**: Stay well-hydrated. Water plays a vital role in maintaining overall health, including cardiovascular function.
- **Physical Activity**: Engage in regular exercise as permitted by your healthcare provider. Aim for activities you enjoy—these could include walking, swimming, or yoga.
- **Manage Stress**: Incorporate relaxation techniques such as meditation, deep breathing, or mindfulness practices to reduce stress, contributing to heart health.
- **Follow Up**: Regular check-ups with your healthcare provider are crucial to monitor heart health and manage risk factors.

While herbal remedies can offer support for heart health, they should complement—not replace—professional medical treatment. This herbal infusion recipe is designed to aid your recovery and promote cardiovascular wellness after a heart attack. Always consult with your healthcare provider before incorporating new remedies into your healing regimen, especially if you've recently experienced a heart event.

76. Herbal Healing for Chronic Stress: A Recipe for Calm

In our fast-paced world, chronic stress has become a common affliction affecting millions. It's often characterized by a relentless feeling of being overwhelmed and can lead to grave health consequences if left unchecked. Rather than solely relying on medication, many are turning to nature's pharmacy for relief. One of the most effective ways to harness the soothing power of herbs is through a simple but potent herbal tea blend.

Understanding Chronic Stress

Chronic stress doesn't just make you feel anxious; it can have profound effects on your physical and mental health. Symptoms may include fatigue, irritability, headaches, digestive issues, and even heart problems. Therefore, finding relief is not just beneficial—it's essential for your overall well-being.

Herbal remedies have been used for centuries in various cultures to promote relaxation and enhance mental clarity. This section will focus on a go-to herbal remedy that can help mitigate the effects of chronic stress: an herbal tea blend that is easy to prepare and delightful to drink.

The Herbal Healing Recipe: Soothing Stress Tea

Ingredients:

- **Chamomile (1 tablespoon dried flowers):** Renowned for its calming effects, chamomile is a natural sedative that helps reduce anxiety and promote better sleep.
- **Lavender (1 teaspoon dried flowers):** With a distinctive fragrance, lavender not only smells divine but also aids in relaxation and stress relief.
- **Lemon Balm (1 tablespoon dried leaves):** A member of the mint family, lemon balm is known to alleviate anxiety and improve mood. Its mild flavor makes it a pleasant addition to any herbal tea.
- **Passionflower (1 teaspoon dried herb):** This beautiful flower has been used in traditional medicine to treat anxiety and improve sleep quality. It has a calming effect on the nervous system.
- **Honey (to taste):** For added sweetness and its own health benefits, honey can enhance the tea's flavor while providing antioxidants.
- **Hot water (2 cups):** The base of our soothing herbal infusion.

Instructions:

1. **Prepare the Herbs:** Gather your dried herbs. You can find them at health food stores or local herbal shops. Chamomile, lavender, lemon balm, and passionflower

can often be purchased as tea blends, though you can also mix your own.

2. **Boil the Water:** Start by boiling 2 cups of water in a kettle. Once it reaches a rolling boil, remove it from the heat.
3. **Steep the Herbs:** In a teapot or heat-resistant container, add the chamomile, lavender, lemon balm, and passionflower. Pour the hot water over the herbs, ensuring they are fully submerged.
4. **Time to Steep:** Cover the pot and allow the herbs to steep for 10-15 minutes. This will allow their beneficial properties to infuse into the water, creating a powerful herbal infusion.
5. **Strain and Sweeten:** Once steeped, strain the tea into your favorite mug. If desired, add honey to taste for added sweetness and health benefits.
6. **Enjoy:** Sip your tea slowly, taking the time to breathe deeply and reflect. Allow the warmth of the drink and the properties of the herbs to wash over you, helping to clear your mind and promote relaxation.

Tips for Enhancing Your Herbal Tea Experience

- **Mindfulness:** As you sip your tea, practice mindfulness. Focus on the present moment, the warmth of the mug in your hands, and the soothing aroma of the herbs. Consider journaling your thoughts or meditating after your tea.

- **Warm Bath:** Pair this herbal tea with a warm bath infused with a few drops of essential oil (like lavender or chamomile) for an altogether calming experience.
- **Routine:** Incorporate this tea into your daily routine—whether as a morning ritual or an evening wind-down routine. Consistency can lead to more profound effects over time.

Chronic stress can feel overwhelming, but nature offers us a wealth of resources to help combat its effects. This herbal tea recipe is a simple yet effective way to incorporate stress-relieving herbs into your daily life. Always remember, though, if you're experiencing severe stress or anxiety, it's essential to consult with a healthcare professional. By engaging with herbal remedies, you not only take steps toward managing your stress but also reconnect with nature's nurturing touch. So brew a cup, relax, and let the calming properties of these herbs work their magic.

Here's to finding your inner peace, one sip at a time!

The Impact of Mental Stress on Physical Health

Mental stress, characterized by emotional strain and pressure, has become an increasingly prevalent issue in modern society, driven by various factors including work demands, personal relationships, and societal expectations. While the psychological effects of stress are widely recognized, the impact of mental stress on physical health is gaining attention within both the scientific community and healthcare sectors.

Mental stress is a common human experience, often triggered by external pressures and internal conflicts. While occasional stress can serve as a motivator, chronic mental stress can lead to adverse health outcomes, creating a complex interplay between psychological and physical health. Historically, the mind and body were viewed as separate entities, but modern research emphasizes their interconnectedness, demonstrating that psychological states can significantly influence physical health.

Mechanisms Linking Stress to Physical Health

1. Neuroendocrine Response

When a person experiences stress, the body activates the hypothalamic-pituitary-adrenal (HPA) axis, resulting in the release of stress hormones, notably cortisol and adrenaline. While these hormones are crucial for the body's "fight or flight" response, prolonged elevation due to chronic stress can lead to various health problems. Chronic cortisol exposure is linked with increased blood sugar levels, immune suppression, and metabolic dysregulation.

2. Inflammatory Response

Chronic stress also correlates with systemic inflammation. Stress can activate pro-inflammatory cytokines, which may contribute to the development or exacerbation of numerous chronic conditions, including cardiovascular diseases, diabetes, and autoimmune disorders. Inflammation is a critical underlying factor in these health concerns, indicating that stress management could lead to better health outcomes.

3. Autonomic Nervous System

The autonomic nervous system (ANS), which regulates involuntary bodily functions, consists of the sympathetic (fight or flight) and parasympathetic (rest and digest) branches. Chronic stress tends to shift the balance toward sympathetic dominance, resulting in increased heart rate, blood pressure, and respiratory rate. Over time, this prolonged sympathetic activation can lead to heightened risks of cardiovascular disease and other stress-related disorders.

Impact on Specific Health Conditions

1. Cardiovascular Health

The relationship between mental stress and cardiovascular health is well documented. Chronic stress can lead to hypertension, increased heart rate, and higher cholesterol levels, all of which are risk factors for heart disease. Studies have shown that individuals with high levels of stress are significantly more likely to experience heart attacks and strokes.

2. Metabolic Disorders

Stress is also a contributing factor to the development of metabolic disorders, including obesity and diabetes. Individuals under stress may engage in unhealthy coping mechanisms, such as overeating, smoking, or substance abuse, leading to weight gain and insulin resistance. Moreover, stress-induced cortisol elevation encourages fat accumulation, particularly visceral fat associated with metabolic dysfunction.

3. Immune System Function

The immune system can be negatively impacted by chronic stress. Initially, stress may boost immune response; however, prolonged stress results in immune suppression, rendering individuals more susceptible to infections and illness. Chronic stress has also been associated with autoimmune diseases, where the immune system mistakenly attacks the body.

4. Musculoskeletal Disorders

The physical manifestation of stress often includes muscle tension, leading to tension-type headaches, neck pain, and back disorders. Chronic pain conditions can be exacerbated by mental stress, creating a vicious cycle of pain and stress perception.

Strategies for Mitigation

1. Stress Management Techniques

Implementing stress management strategies is crucial for mitigating the effects of mental stress on physical health. Techniques such as mindfulness meditation, progressive muscle relaxation, and yoga can significantly reduce stress levels and enhance overall well-being.

2. Physical Activity

Regular physical activity is a powerful tool for combating stress. Exercise not only reduces muscular tension but also promotes the release of endorphins, which are known to improve mood and reduce perceptions of pain and stress.

3. Social Support

Building robust social networks can serve as a buffer against stress. Support from family, friends, or community can provide emotional assistance and contribute to resilience against stressors.

4. Professional Help

Engaging with mental health professionals can offer therapeutic avenues to cope with stress. Cognitive-behavioral therapy (CBT) and other counseling modalities have proven effective in helping individuals manage stress and its health impacts.

The Connection between Our Emotions, Mental Health, and Physical Well-Being

As we traverse the intricate maze of life, we often encounter ups and downs that shape our emotional landscapes. Our emotions do not exist in a vacuum; they are intimately intertwined with our mental health and physical well-being. Understanding this connection is essential, as it allows us to develop healthier coping strategies and foster better overall health.

Understanding Emotions

Emotions are complex reactions that involve physiological, cognitive, and behavioral responses to internal and external stimuli. They serve as our body's early warning system—alerting us to danger, excitement, sadness, or any number of states we may feel.

"The body experience is linked to the emotional experience—in times of stress, we become physically tense or fatigued; in times of joy, we may feel energized or light," — *Dr. Susan David, Psychologist and Author.*

Recognizing our emotions is the first step in understanding how they influence our mental and physical health.

The Link between Emotions and Mental Health

Our emotional state has a profound effect on our mental health. Here are some ways in which emotions and mental health are connected:

1. **Emotional Resilience**: Emotions help us respond to life's challenges. When we cultivate emotional resilience, we can better handle stress, reducing the likelihood of mental health issues such as anxiety and depression.
2. **Cognitive Function**: Negative emotions can impair cognitive functions like memory, attention, and decision-making. Conversely, positive emotions enhance our cognitive capabilities, promoting mental clarity.
3. **Social Connections**: Our emotional states affect how we interact with others. Positive emotions create stronger bonds, while negative emotions can strain relationships, further exacerbating mental health issues.
4. **Stress Response**: Emotions related to stress, such as anxiety and frustration, can trigger the body's fight or flight response. Over time, chronic stress can lead to more severe mental health problems.

Strategies for Enhancing Emotional Health

Understanding the connections we've discussed, let's consider some actionable steps we can take to enhance our emotional health, which in turn supports our overall mental and physical health:

1. **Practice Mindfulness**: Engaging in mindfulness practices such as meditation or yoga can help us become more aware of our emotions and reduce symptoms of anxiety and depression.
2. **Seek Connection**: Building and maintaining social connections can provide emotional support and create a sense of belonging, which is vital for mental health.
3. **Physical Activity**: Regular exercise helps to reduce stress and improve mood through the release of endorphins, promoting both emotional and physical well-being.
4. **Healthy Coping Mechanisms**: Find healthy outlets for expressing and processing emotions, such as journaling, art, or talking to a therapist.
5. **Eat Balanced Meals**: Nutrition plays a crucial role in our emotional health. A balanced diet rich in fruits, vegetables, whole grains, and healthy fats can help stabilize mood.
6. **Adequate Sleep**: Prioritize sleep hygiene to ensure that we are well-rested; a good night's sleep is essential for both emotional regulation and overall health.

FAQs

Q1: How do emotions contribute to stress-related illnesses?

A1: Emotions such as chronic anxiety and anger can lead to prolonged stress, which in turn can cause physical ailments like hypertension and heart disease.

Q2: Can emotional health be improved through therapy?

A2: Yes, therapy can provide tools to manage emotions effectively, offering strategies to enhance emotional resilience and overall health.

Q3: What role does diet play in emotional health?

A3: A well-balanced diet rich in micronutrients can influence neurotransmitter function, leading to better mood regulation and emotional stability.

Q4: Are there physical symptoms of emotional distress?

A4: Yes, emotional distress may manifest physically as headaches, digestive issues, or unexplained aches and pains.

Q5: How can I tell if my emotions are impacting my health?

A5: If you notice increased stress-related symptoms, changes in your sleeping patterns, or unwarranted physical pain, it's essential to evaluate your emotional health.

In overall, accepting a deeper understanding of the relationship between our emotions, mental health, and general physical well-being is crucial. As we become more attuned to our emotional landscape, we better equip ourselves to handle life's challenges effectively. By implementing practical strategies to enhance our emotional health, we can improve not only our mental health but also our physical health, creating a holistic approach to well-being that is both sustainable and transformative.

BE WELL!

THE POWER OF HEALING HERBS

www.ingramcontent.com/pod-product-compliance
Lightning Source LLC
Chambersburg PA
CBHW061621250726
48659CB00004B/1028